100
SIMPLE SECRETS
OF
GREAT
RELATIONSHIPS

Also in this series

100
SIMPLE SECRETS
OF
GREAT
RELATIONSHIPS

WHAT SCIENTISTS HAVE LEARNED
AND HOW YOU CAN USE IT

DAVID NIVEN, Ph.D.

HarperSanFrancisco
A Division of HarperCollins*Publishers*

HarperCollins books may be purchased for educational, business, or sales promotional use. For information please write: Special Markets Department, HarperCollins Publishers, 10 East 53rd Street, New York, NY 10022.

HarperCollins Web site: http://www.harpercollins.com

HarperCollins®, ☒®, and HarperSanFrancisco™
are trademarks of HarperCollins Publishers.

FIRST EDITION

Library of Congress Cataloging-in-Publication Data is available.
ISBN-13: 978-0-06-115790-5
ISBN-10: 0-06-115790-2

06 07 08 09 10 CW 10 9 8 7 6 5 4 3 2 1

Contents

A Note to Readers

Each of the 100 entries presented here is based on the research conclusions of scientists studying relationships. Each entry contains a key research finding complemented by advice and an example following from the finding. The research conclusions presented in each entry are based on a meta-analysis of research on relationships, which means that each conclusion is derived from the work of multiple researchers studying the same topic. To enable the reader to find further information on each topic, a reference to a supporting study is included in each entry, and a bibliography of recent work on relationships has also been provided.

http://www.iciba.com/

Introduction

I was speaking to a group of senior citizens gathered in a community recreation center in Delray Beach, Florida. In the audience there must have been at least two dozen people who had been married for three decades or more. They had seen the full spectrum of relationships—and heard the full spectrum of relationship advice. After my talk they asked what I was currently working on, and I mentioned I was studying research conclusions on relationships. Now the comments were flying in.

The seniors disagreed about a number of points, but they all nodded yes when one man said, "There's no topic out there with more bad advice. Well, maybe the stock market, but it's up there. Top two, definitely." Stories came forward from couples married forty and fifty years about having been told by friends their marriage wouldn't last six months. Another said her mother told her on her wedding day she didn't think she would be married six weeks later.

"There aren't any songs about young people being encouraged by their friends and family to spend their lives together—they're all about warnings," one woman said. "It's all how hard and terrible it will be. It will never last. That's because relationships are the one thing everyone is a naysayer about when it comes to everybody else's situation.

"Now, there wouldn't be any relationships if people applied this thinking to themselves. Personally, they have to be optimists. 'Of course things will work out.' But with somebody else, it's always, 'I don't know; it will be tough. Are you sure you're ready?'"

While they shared a skepticism about bad advice—advice that comes from people who are angry at the world or who want someone to commiserate with—they admitted they were apt to share their own views with their children, grandchildren, and sometimes just about anyone.

But their comments were generally spoken with an air of optimism and promise regarding their own relationships—an optimism that was in stark contrast to the negative words they heard as younger men and women. Among the points they told me I should include in my book were

- Find a happy medium, which includes some time together and some time alone.
- Have patience, communication, and compromise.
- Talk out any problems that arise.
- Be unselfish.
- Have a strong work ethic, a sense of humor, and a love of family.
- Say "I'm sorry," "thank you," and "I forgot."
- Have mutual respect.
- Enjoy each other's company.
- Work together for the true, the good, and the beautiful.
- Respect each other's integrity, and understand differences.
- Show your appreciation for each other.
- Say, "in sickness and in health, but never for lunch."
- Always say good night even if you are still upset about something.

While I explained that I would be working from the findings of scientific studies on relationships, the seniors told me I could come back anytime for more of their advice.

The *100 Simple Secrets of Great Relationships* presents the conclusions of scientists who have studied the relationships, dating habits, and marriages of millions of people. Each entry presents the core scientific finding, a real-world example of the principle, and the basic advice you should follow to increase satisfaction with your personal life.

As I conducted the research for this book, combing through thousands of reports on relationships, I saw studies confirming many of the ideas the folks at the senior center had shared with me. And while the world around us has changed in innumerable ways since they were married, the core realities of human need for relationships and what humans need from relationships remain. And, in a great comfort to my friends at the senior center, these findings are not pessimistic. The great thrust of the research that has been done, and that I write about here, is completely in keeping with the wisdom of one of the gentlemen at the senior center, who said, "It takes effort. It isn't easy. But anyone can do it. I mean, look at me, for example."

The Mundane Is Heroic

Some tasks we think of as difficult and their achievement noteworthy. Others we think of as boring and their achievement insignificant. Of course, the tasks that are noteworthy are often built on a foundation of the mundane. Firefighters study lifesaving techniques and firefighting protocols for years on end, and then one day they are called on to use their skills and knowledge to save a building and the people in it. Without the years of mundane commitment, there would be no moment of great achievement. We recognize that having a long-standing healthy relationship is an achievement. If you are married long enough, the local newspaper will take your picture and write up your story. But that achievement is built on a nearly infinite series of actions, including a daily, hourly, moment-to-moment commitment to each other. It is certainly not always easy, and the rewards are not always immediately apparent, but sacrificing your immediate preferences and being committed to sharing, caring, and listening are mundane but heroic steps toward your lifetime relationship goal.

EVEN BEFORE they dated, Kathy and William began working out together. Later, after they married, their interest and success in running led them to set a goal of running together in the Boston Marathon. After training for three years together working toward that goal, Kathy's best time qualified her for the race and William's did not.

William could have reacted in a variety of ways, all of them perfectly normal, given human nature. He could have wallowed in self-pity, dragging both himself and his wife down and making her feel somehow guilty for his exclusion. He could have asked Kathy to wait until they could run together. He could have resented his wife's ability to achieve and tried to sabotage her. [ˈsæbətɑːʒ]

"A big part of me wished I was out there running the marathon, of course," admitted William. "So what did I do on race day? I went out to five or six locations and cheered her on." William chose to encourage rather than discourage. "I lived vicariously through her. Her success is my success."

William says that in working out together, as in life together, jealousy, [ˈdʒeləsi] envy, and other unpleasant emotions can visit relationships, but the most important thing to remember is that "we're a team every day—race day, too. We have to be able to give each other the freedom to be able to develop our own talents. To not stand in each other's way, but to stand with each other, helping if we can, watching if we can't."

The ability to maintain open, healthy communication in a relationship is associated with strong levels of such highly regarded personal qualities as self-restraint, courage, generosity, commitment to justice, and good judgment. (Fowers 2001)

See Possibilities Where Others See Obstacles

In any relationship, it is possible to find evidence that suggests the relationship will thrive or evidence that predicts it just won't work. Even the strongest, best relationships experience problems that suggest it might not last. And even in the most tenuous relationships, there are reasons to think it just might work well. The real question is which evidence you pay more attention to. Constant attention to the weaknesses of any relationship will weaken it. Constant attention to the strengths of any relationship will strengthen it.

IT IS PERHAPS the ultimate example of love and devotion trumping religious differences and the associated political differences: Pam is Jewish, Adil is Muslim, and they have been happily married for more than a decade.

Adil explains the effort it takes to keep his world in order: "When I am with my mother I say 'we' about the Muslims, and when I am here with my wife I say 'we' about the Jews. Sometimes I stop and don't know what to say—'we, they.'"

"The political issues can go on and on," Pam sighed. "But I always like to take things back to our lives, to here and now."

When they met, Adil was interested in asking Pam out on a date but worried she might not want to be involved with a Muslim. "I remember this tension, thinking if I should tell her right away that I am a Muslim," he recalled.

[əˈblɪviəs]

"I wasn't oblivious and I was well aware of the differences," she said. "But I thought I had the courage to manage." While both sets of parents were ultimately supportive, the society Adil and Pam chose to inhabit wasn't.

"People are so intense," said Pam. "Everywhere you go it is Jew, Arab, Arab, Jew. You can't just be." There have been many double takes, criticisms, and insults. Too many to count.

Determined and in love, Adil and Pam have worked to straddle the distance between Jewish and Muslim cultures, to exist in the open. In [ˈdɪstəmɪn] the meantime, symbols and sounds of coexistence permeate their home. [ɑːmˈwɑːɪ] Their dining room armoire displays a Koran next to a menorah. The fam- 大型衣櫥 ily celebrates Jewish holidays alongside Muslim ones. [məˈnɔːrə]

"It is possible for this to work," Pamela said. "A committed couple can survive. If we had considered only the difficulties, we would have nothing. But we saw past them, and now we have everything that matters."

"If there is anything our relationship might suggest about how our two worlds can get along, it is compromise," Adil said. "It's the magic word."

[ˈkɔmprəmaɪz]

❋

In an experiment performed with couples who were experiencing conflict, [ˈkɔnflɪkt] half of the couples were asked to discuss the best part of their relationship and half to discuss the worst aspect of their relationship. Couples discussing the positive side of their relationship reduced their stress level by 15 percent, while couples discussing the negative side saw their stress level increase 48 percent. (Sullivan 2001)

4

Set Rules for Conflict

While every relationship has disagreements, the number and severity of those disagreements vary tremendously. You are never going to agree on everything, and you shouldn't try to agree on everything. But one vital agreement will help you reduce the pain of disagreements: choosing a method for your discussions. It is not uncommon to find two people in a relationship with wildly different ideas about how to deal with conflict. Some rush into it the first moment they notice the problem, others hint around the problem without directly stating it, and still others try to avoid the subject and perhaps the instigating event altogether. The real problem arises when two people in a relationship adopt different approaches. Now not only do they have to deal with the conflict at hand, but the difference in their approaches alone causes tension. Level the playing field in your discussions by deciding how you can air concerns to each other in a format that allows both of you to participate.

JAMES LEIJA KNOWS a thing or two about conflict. He's a professional boxer, among the best in the lightweight class. "Although I box, I hit people. I do it within the rules. You have to have rules—or you have no sport."

He lives his life by the same standard. James and his wife, Lisa, were high school sweethearts before getting married. They have no wedding day photos because James was still black and blue from U.S. Olympic boxing trials on the big day. Now, in addition to his career, they focus on raising their children and the family dog (a boxer named Knuckles).

The first years were lean. James turned pro but barely made enough money to pay for his training expenses. Lisa worked as a receptionist and paid for everything else. They drove a beat-up car. "We never once fought about money because we both agreed there were more important things in life," Lisa says. "But it was rough."

Finally James told his manager, Lester Bedford, that he could no longer afford to keep boxing. Bedford begged him to reconsider and gave Lisa $250 for Christmas. The Leijas persevered, month to month, fight to fight, hoping for a break.

The break finally came with a fight against a top contender and, when James won, a bout against the champion. By the time he had claimed the world junior lightweight title, he was rich beyond his imagination. "It's like we're living out a book," Lisa says. "You can hardly wait to see what's going to happen next. We have an awesome story. We didn't hide from each other. We faced our fears and our hard times together."

Now, instead of money worries, they have to deal with groupies. "Girls just threw themselves at him during autograph sessions," manager Lester recalls. Before they could argue over it, James thought about Lisa's feelings and decided to avoid places where he would draw too much attention.

"This is a sport where divorce is as common as blood in the ring," Lester says. "But James and Lisa have figured out how to put each other first."

While people may employ many different conflict resolution strategies in a relationship, when both partners use the same strategy they experience 12 percent less conflict and are 31 percent more likely to report their relationship is satisfying. (Pape 2001)

Anyone Can Find a Happy Relationship

Describe the kinds of people you think are destined for a happy relationship. What kind of work do they do? How old are they? How much money do they make? How much education do they have? What religion are they? You probably have some pretty strong images in your mind. But the truth is that none of these factors determines relationship quality. People of every kind of background have found happiness in relationships, and people of every kind of background have encountered difficulties. Fulfilling relationships have everything to do with who you are but not with what you are.

RICK WORKS for the forestry service in Wyoming. He says his unit is stationed halfway between the middle of nowhere and not much else. In the tiny isolated towns in the area, there are few men and even fewer women.

"I still have hope that I'll find the right woman, and I'm holding out for that," says Rick, who is thirty-two and unmarried. "It's not just a fantasy. I believe there's something like a soul mate out there, something close to that true connection, that feeling when you know you can't live without this other person and you don't want to. But at the same time it's scary. What if I don't find her?

"I don't expect everything today," he continues. "There aren't very many women out here, but I know what I am and what I've done will be interesting to people—and when I'm back in the world I know someone will want to find out more."

He concludes, "I'm not working on a deadline—I'm not a product on the shelf that's going to expire. I'm going to live my life and find someone. I have no doubt. Look around you at the evidence—all sorts of people are finding each other all the time, all over the place. I'll find the right person for me."

Age, income, education, and religion are unrelated to the likelihood of relationship satisfaction. (Koehne 2000)

It's Not How Hard You Try

I'm going to work on my relationship."

"I'm going to put my all into it."

We've heard platitudes about hard work all our lives. But trying really hard, by itself, is not a recipe for success. In fact, maximum effort can be a great source of frustration and pain when our efforts are not rewarded with a better relationship. Work on your relationship with meaningful goals that will contribute to your relationship's health and your happiness. Work on your relationship with logic and reason, not with maximum effort.

NICOLE HAD PICTURED this day almost her entire life. It was all she had thought about for months. Everything she did was focused on it. It was to be a picture-perfect wedding.

The flowers had been imported from New Zealand. The reception was planned for the Grand Salon of the Essex House in Manhattan. Nicole was wearing a stunning Cristoff-designed wedding gown, with a four-karat diamond ring glistening on her left hand.

Everything was set on the wedding day. Except for one small detail: Nicole's fiancé had already left for their Tahitian honeymoon. Without her. The bride's mother watched "as a beautiful wedding turned into a nightmare." Nicole soldiered on and attended the reception party for the nonwedding and then went about putting her world back in order.

Friends quietly wondered if the wedding fiasco wasn't a case of trying too hard. "Sometimes people see marriage differently. They see their relationship to one another differently. One may think she's being open and honest in professing her love and pushing the relationship, but the other may just feel pushed," said a friend. "She needed to pace the relationship. You can go too fast and try too hard."

People who said they were trying hard to improve their relationship were 33 percent less likely to be happy than were people who said they were putting some effort into improving their relationship. (Hairston 2001)

You Have Nothing to Envy

If you were thinking about potential partners, you would no doubt be excited about finding someone who was very successful at work. And yet in a relationship, people often find themselves envious of the success of their partner. They begin to see the success of their partner as a personal failure or as a score in some kind of competition. This makes little sense and does no one any good. There is no trophy for bettering your partner. The real prize goes to those who refuse to compete with their partner. That prize is contentment and a more satisfying relationship.

WHEN GEORGE BURNS and Gracie Allen first teamed up onstage to perform a comedy act in the 1930s, he had the experience and she was new to the business. George took the lead and had Gracie feed him the straight lines while he told all the jokes. The act was a disaster. "The trained seal got more applause," Burns said.

The next night George took the straight lines and gave Gracie all the laugh lines. The rest is show business history. Or as George put it, "I asked Gracie about her brother, and she talked for the next thirty-eight years."

First onstage, then on radio, and then on TV, the real-life and stage couple played their roles to the hilt, she a befuddled wife, he an exasperated husband. All the while, Gracie was the center of attention, telling the jokes while George worked the setups for her lines.

For George Burns, standing out of the spotlight in the act while his wife was the center of the show was simply a recognition of ability. "Gracie had a talent the audience loved. I had a talent the audience didn't. I knew how to write it, and she knew how to say it.

"Gracie got all the laughs," he added, "and that was all right with me, because we split the salaries, and that was good, too."

Married for four decades until Gracie passed away, George Burns always wanted her recognized as the star of the show. "Gracie should always have top billing," he said.

People who feel a sense of competition with their partner are 37 percent less likely to feel that their relationship is satisfying. (Romero-Medina 2001)

Attitude Triumphs over Outcome

People can get discouraged easily. We want something badly, and when we can't seem to get it we can lose hope. But the world is changing every day. You are changing every day. There is no way to predict exactly what will happen or when it will happen. What you can do is continue. Continue being someone who contributes to others' happiness. Continue being someone who sees the good around you. Continue being someone who would offer love, affection, and support to the right partner.

ELLEN HAS LIVED and worked in New York City for almost a decade. She says looking for a relationship in the city can be harder than finding a seat on the subway at rush hour.

"Everyone has their guard up, and everybody has a busy schedule and an agenda. It is sometimes hard to just relax and meet someone.

"There's not a lot of warmth because people are in a hurry," Ellen says. "People are putting in long hours, and it's hard to make a transition to being social. People are defensive. If you try to approach a stranger, the reaction is, 'Who are you? Are you normal?'"

Ellen has not given up; in fact, she's convinced things can only get better. "Five years ago, I was getting pretty serious with a guy I was dating. I trusted him. After we dated a few months, he told the building manager he was my husband, and they gave him the key to my apartment.

"He took jewelry and camera equipment, found the keys to my car, and drove my stuff away in it."

Fortunately for Ellen, he also stole one more thing. "He took a pair of concert tickets. They were really good seats. That's how the cops found him—in my seats at a rock concert at Madison Square Garden. With another woman.

"I'm glad I have a positive outlook. I get a good laugh out of all this. I don't let it bother me; I just keep on dating."

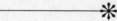

In long-term studies of people over the course of multiple decades, the capacity to ultimately find a happy relationship was not affected by the age when they first fell in love. But it was affected by the person's attitude toward their experiences. (Werner and Smith 2001)

Don't Be Bound by Tradition

How many times have we heard a parent, grandparent, or other senior person tell us about how they did things in their day? We have so much exposure to some traditional ideas and behaviors that we are almost forced to assume that they are both important and reasonable. In reality, over time the patterns in relationships have been evolving dramatically. For a relationship to function and thrive, we must live within our own standards, not those imposed from another time.

JAIME THOUGHT he was a good husband and father. He worked long days, but his work paid for life's necessities. On days off his attitude was "Don't bother me."

He remembers the ominous feeling in the pit of his stomach when his own father used to come home late from work. "It never seemed like he wanted to be there with my mom and us." Yet, Jaime was ashamed to admit, he seemed to be repeating the cycle.

Jaime says that his experience is all too common. "The story my friends tell all the time is that they saw their own dads just going to work. That was the role of the man. The role of the woman was to keep tabs on the kids. Latino dads find it hard to express positive emotion—to tell their wife how important she is or to tell their kids they are making you proud.

"Finally I cut the circle. I said no more. I want my wife and children to come to me, to be happy when I come home."

Jaime's new perspective came with his involvement in Los Padres, a Colorado-based group of Latino dads devoted to improving communication with their wives and children. They hold classes and regular meetings to share a message of family commitment.

"In Los Padres, we are redefining *macho*. Being a real man, a family man, means communicating, not wanting to be left alone. Being a man means getting down on the floor and playing with your child. It means never being afraid to show love."

Jaime's involvement in Los Padres has changed his life and his family's life. "I appreciate what great gifts have been given to me, and I make sure my family knows that. And with Los Padres, I'm helping to make sure other men in this community see what they have. Not just their obligations, but their hope."

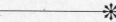

Studies of relationships find that in the last two decades both men's and women's expectations have changed significantly and become less rigid. Today, partners in happy, long-term relationships are three times more likely to embrace a flexible definition of women's and men's roles. (Gilbert and Walker 2001)

The Past Is Not the Future

If you wanted to predict the weather, you could look at past weather patterns, and you would get a pretty good idea of the temperatures and the rainy season. The past would be a good indicator of the future. The same is not true for your relationships. Your relationship history is not your relationship future. Your relationship future is not limited by your experiences of the past or by your disappointments of the past. You can't change the weather, but you can change your relationship pattern; you can learn from your experiences and avoid mistakes of the past.

MONICA SELES KNOWS she will always be measured against her younger self, the one who turned tennis professional at fifteen and swept past Steffi Graf to claim the number one ranking a little more than two years later.

She practiced relentlessly. She was fearless. She was ranked number one for 178 weeks. In an astounding four-year run, from 1990 to 1993, she won eight of the twelve Grand Slam titles. And what, really, did it get her?

"Money, titles—those are all great, and as an athlete you practice really hard to get that. It doesn't mean it's going to make you happy. As a child, you think it's that way—'I'm going to make my first million bucks; that's what will make me happy.' It will definitely give you a sense of security and a lot of things, but that's not going to make you happy."

That sense of security was of little solace after a deranged man burst from the stands and stabbed her in the back during a break in her match in the 1993 German Open.

"I got stopped at the height of my career," Seles said. "A lot of things could have been different. It was very hard for me to get going again." Her power—after the stabbing and a chronic shoulder injury—and quickness diminished. But she has persevered to reclaim a place among the best players in the world. Even after climbing all the way back, she admits the deep desire is no longer there on a daily basis.

"I've learned not to stake my happiness on a tennis match. Every day you play, you win some, you lose some. If you treat people based on how you did on the tennis court, which a lot of players do, you'll wind up throwing away your personal life. If your emotions depend on tennis, you're going to be a nervous wreck. My life has gone through ups and downs, but I think that happens to everybody. My theory is you get up and try again in every way, in every aspect of life—in your career, in your personal life. You just keep going on."

Seles embraces the notion that she can make a positive change in her life. "I don't believe you can ever be what you were in the past because of so many things, your experiences," she said. "You cannot be the same person. I live in the present. There is no other way, because you cannot worry about the past or the future."

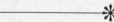

Most people who exited an unhappy relationship were in a happy relationship within three years, and 74 percent said that their new relationship was significantly different. (Sweeney 2002)

No One Wins the Comparison Game

Logically, our personal life doesn't change when we compare it to the relationships our friends have. But the way we think about it does. Thus when we see a friend or family member enjoying a seemingly perfect relationship, we begin to question our own. Or if we see a friend or family member struggling in a relationship, it makes us think better of our own. Don't let yourself play this comparison game. Your relationship must be evaluated based on your own needs, not on the relative relationship success of those around you.

IT IS A RELATIONSHIP with a storybook start. Two friends from college promise to write to each other when the marines call him off to active duty in the Gulf War. Their letters go from friendly to intimate. Another letter from a military camp in Saudi Arabia contains a marriage proposal.

More than a decade later, Tim and Karen both have been back to school for another degree, and they have three children. And that means romance has had to share a crowded decade with morning sickness, graduate research projects, and stretches where a new CD was a splurge.

"Years two through four were volatile," Tim remembers. "Any little thing could set us off," Karen agreed. "When you're young, everything is about you."

"A piece of us was just stubborn enough that we fought through some things," Tim says. "We just hung in there."

When times were at their worst, Tim fell back on his training for a business degree. "I began to think about how tough I had it, how people I knew seemed to be getting along much better. Then I thought about what I'd been taught in some of my business and marketing courses—that we have a consumer mentality. Anything from a long-distance phone company to a VCR can be replaced if it stops meeting our needs. And I saw that people can do that to their relationship. I was doing that to my relationship—treating it as a product and wondering if I couldn't trade it in for a better one.

"If you think about a relationship as a consumer, if you start comparing your spouse to others, then you've undermined what you have for what probably doesn't exist. After all, marketing is about making us dislike what we have and think what someone else has is better."

Tim says when he realized he wasn't keeping score on his marriage, "I was free to put my energy into it, instead of putting my energy into wondering whether this was worth it."

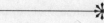

People who were asked first to describe an unhappy couple then to describe their own relationship were 19 percent more likely to describe their relationship enthusiastically than were people who were first asked to describe a happy couple and then describe their own relationship. (Carsten 2001)

See the Love Around You

We are sometimes quick to see the problems in our lives and reluctant to see the strengths of our lives. Regardless of your relationship status, think of the many people who love you and the depth of their love for you. Feeling loved and knowing that you are worthy of love are necessary to creating or maintaining any relationship.

LANCE AND REBECCA were already married with a son when Lance enrolled in law school. A professor warned that the law school grind had ended more marriages than he could count. In fact, three years later Lance was the only student in his graduating class still married to the same person. Lance and Rebecca both admit, however, that those years were "terrible."

"There were days when he'd go to school and I'd just cry," Rebecca said. "I felt like Lance was in law school and I was knee-deep in changing diapers, but that there wasn't really a 'we.'"

Their relationship continued in a state of wedded mediocrity after law school. Then eight years later a doctor told Rebecca she had a terminal disease.

"I started withdrawing and preparing for her death," Lance said. "I couldn't comprehend living without her. I withdrew, even though that's when Rebecca needed me more than ever. I got colder. I couldn't face life without her." They didn't communicate; they didn't know how to reach out.

"I didn't want anything fixed. I wanted to be hugged and held," Rebecca remembers. "But I figured out that it was fear, not lack of love, that was causing Lance to run away."

Eventually, another doctor caught the misdiagnosis. Rebecca's health improved dramatically when she stopped taking the medicine that had been making her sick. The emotional healing, however, took longer.

"For me, it's letting go of resentments and scars for the years when I felt alone and then when I thought I was dying," she said. "I don't look back. What we are doing today keeps the relationship growing. I know I'm loved, and I will always be loved. And Lance is trying harder to show it in all kinds of ways."

Lance thinks he understands her needs better now. "Rebecca has always been there for me. To me, that is the definition of romance. To love so much that you are always there. She made me feel loved. I see that I can do more of that so that we're in it together."

People do not experience love in isolation from their other personal relationships. For example, people in satisfying relationships were 22 percent more likely to think of themselves as well loved by family members and friends than were people with unsatisfying relationships. (Sprecher and Felmlee 2000)

Doing Nothing Is Rarely a Solution

When we don't have an answer, or when we don't like the answer, it is often tempting to ignore the problem. Ignoring the problem may help you this moment, but it is not a solution. You can ignore problems only so long, until they grow far larger and far harder to solve. Approach your relationship with all your attention and abilities, the way you would approach anything that is important to you.

"YOU MAY NOT find this on too many greeting cards, but the fact of the matter is that it's not love but arguing that is pivotal to happy marriages," says Professor David Olson. Olson has made a career of studying relationships, and he adds, "After all, we know that all couples who marry are in love. Yet 50 percent of them divorce. And the biggest predictor of staying together is how well they're able to work through their differences."

Professor Olson says people need to understand that thoughtful love and careful conflict are two sides of the same coin. "Loving well builds up reservoirs of fondness that help couples get through tough times; arguing well avoids the kind of scorched-earth disagreements that drain that reservoir dry."

But Professor Olson worries that too many couples slight the disagreement part, hurting their shot at happiness. And that concern inspired him to create a protocol among counselors that involves relationship questionnaires—to find likely sore spots—and then step-by-step lessons on how to talk problems out.

His records are impressive. Olson can predict with 85 percent accuracy which of the engaged couples who fill out his questionnaire will split up within three years. And in a five-year field study, couples cut their risk of divorce by two-thirds by following the program's lessons in communication and conflict resolution.

Laurie and Dave are one couple who took Professor Olson's test and received follow-up counseling. They credit it with making their relationship stronger. Laurie said she constantly avoided conflict in previous relationships. "This was a big issue in my first marriage," she said. "We always had to have a winner and a loser. So I'd get scared of disagreements and basically run and hide from them."

Laurie's apprehension registered on her, so she and Dave worked on that in sessions with a marriage and family therapist. "Dave worked to reassure me there were other options besides mega-arguments," Laurie said. Now, when Dave senses her withdrawing, he'll coax her to talk rather than clam up. "And I think we both help each other stay on track with whatever we're talking about—money, religion, whatever."

Married couples who report they never argue with each other are 35 percent more likely to divorce within four years than are couples who report regularly disagreeing. (Vaughn 2001)

You'll Forget the Disagreement but Remember the Disagreeing

T hink of the disagreements you've had with your partner in the past six months. They blend together, don't they? Who left what where, who did this, who forgot to do that? It all can seem quite fuzzy after a while. Now try to remember how you felt during those disagreements. It's much, much easier to remember that, isn't it? You might have felt belittled, or you might have felt disappointed, or perhaps, ultimately, you felt that your opinion was respected. The point is that we remember the atmosphere, the feelings of a disagreement, long after we forget the specifics of the disagreement. Regardless of the disagreement at hand, remember to always put the feelings of your partner ahead of the specific complaint because the feelings will linger long after the complaint is solved or forgotten.

HE SELLS CARS for a living. She sells cars for a living. Adam and Sandra are both blessed with the gift of gab, with a confidence that they will get what they want when they speak to anyone. And how does that work in their relationship? "Well, you can finish each other's jokes. Because you know all the same lines."

When disagreements come up, though, both admit their personalities could be a problem. "If you look at it in terms of expecting to get what you want, this could be a disaster," Adam says. "But if you look at it from the perspective that we are two people used to seeing things through somebody else's point of view, it is really a strength."

"Our trade is really about understanding," Sandra agrees. "Understanding what people are looking for and what they are all about. In our relationship, it really helps us to see what the other person is saying. We respect each other, and each other's needs, so when we disagree we really get to the heart of the matter about what is wrong, what the other person needs."

What about the add-ons, floor mats, CD players, and tinted windows that they artfully suggest after the huge sticker price has been absorbed? "Well, we can't really get away with anything when we know each other's moves. More importantly, you can't take advantage of someone twice. People may not remember the exact details, but they remember how you treated them. We know that. We have to be ready to make our commitment and stick to it. In the end we find a lot more things to agree on than to disagree on."

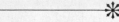

Asked to describe three recent disagreements with their partner, people had ten times as much to say about their feelings and the tone of the disagreement as about the topic of the disagreement. Twenty-five percent of people forgot the topic of a disagreement but could describe their feelings on the situation. (Ludwig 2000)

Pursue What You Need Forever,
Not What You Want Today

We are happy when we get what we want and unhappy when we don't get what we want. Aren't we? Actually, we are happy when we get what we want only if what we want serves our needs. In other words, getting exactly what we want every minute would be like a child getting a candy bar every time she desires one. She may be happy eating the first one, but over time she'll grow tired of candy and have rotten teeth. View the search for a happy relationship not as a process of immediate satisfaction but as a means to pursue your fundamental needs.

BRENDA AND MARTY are dedicated to each other and to the children they serve in state-run children's services agencies. Unfortunately, they work for different states.

While they can't see each other every day, they email each other several times a day. "Generally we send messages to each other every morning. Every night after work we check messages, and sometimes we're on together. And then before I go to bed each night, I say good night. Usually there are three messages a day, back and forth. We talk about our days, our work, our dogs.

"Regardless of how well you know a person, and how long you have lived with that person, I think corresponding with them shows you a completely different side of them," Brenda says. "A letter, even an email, is like a window into their soul. I think I know him better now than when I lived every day with him. Since the beginning of time, men have gone off to war or sailed the seas or found various other ways to make a living that have forced them to live away from their loved ones. The letters they would write would frequently be full of warmth and feeling, and our email is no different." Fortunately, they've yet to have an online argument.

Brenda and Marty do spend every other weekend together. "The weekends we're together are like honeymoons. We spend lots of time doing fun things. I think most married folks don't devote two entire weekends a month to their relationships like we do," Brenda says.

Marty readily admits, "Living apart isn't always easy. I speak for us both when I say that we would rather be living together. I'm very proud of Brenda and what she has accomplished. It's important to both of us that she pursue her career, even if it means some time away from each other. For me, it's fun to travel to see her."

"Marty is the most wonderful husband," says Brenda. "He has always been supportive of everything I do, even when I have wild ideas, like taking a job in another state. We are partners."

"But, this life is not for everyone," Marty says. "You have to believe and trust your partner. You have to spend quality, nurturing, and loving time together. I think a lot of marriages don't work because living together on a daily basis is very difficult. We appreciate each other more because of the time we spend apart. It's a joy to be together because it's a rare and special treat. We have a wonderful life together."

Brenda adds a caution about the bottom line: "A long-distance relationship takes two people who respect each other's needs and who want to make it work."

Couples that pursue a hedonistic form of happiness, seeking to fulfill their desires regardless of their needs, endure twice as much conflict as couples that pursue more altruistic forms of happiness (that is, based on creating feelings of unity and mutual satisfaction). (Loveless 2000)

15

Seek Harmony in Your Life

If our personal life is tough, we think about retreating to our workplace, where we will find satisfaction. If our job is unsatisfying, we think about escaping to our personal life, where we will find fulfillment. In truth, we tend to carry with us the feelings from one part of our life into the other. If part of our life is not working, then we will carry that pain into everything else we do. A satisfying life is not one in which you feel good about one part of your life and ignore the other parts, but one in which you feel rewarded in everything you care about.

ACTRESS SONDRA LOCKE starred in *The Heart Is a Lonely Hunter*, which earned her an Oscar nomination. Then she appeared in a series of films (*The Outlaw Josey Wales, Every Which Way but Loose, Bronco Billy, Any Which Way You Can,* and *Sudden Impact*) starring Clint Eastwood.

A romance began with the first picture they worked on together, in 1975. The chemistry was instant. "He was more than handsome," she said. "He was compelling. In spite of all the usual bustle and chaos on a movie set, there was a hushed aura surrounding him, like the quiet at the center of a storm. Just as he was about to look away into the distant desert, he caught sight of me. I wasn't prepared for the way our eyes seemed to instantly fuse."

He invited her to dinner. She accepted. They became inseparable. He bought them a wonderful country property in northern California.

The star frowned on her interest in expanding her acting career outside his movies. She let her career go—at first appearing only in his movies and then not appearing in any movies. "I didn't think about it initially, but three years in, I saw it." Locke understood that if she pursued her own career, "it would be at the risk of our relationship. And when I did, that was the beginning of the end.

"Certainly I take responsibility for it. I let the relationship be a substitute for my career. And instead of finding joy in both, I wound up with neither."

Researchers find a spillover effect such that people who experience high levels of conflict in their relationship are 20 percent less satisfied with their job, and people who experience high levels of stress on the job are 38 percent less satisfied with their personal life. (Ludlow and Alvarez-Salvat 2001)

16

The Relationship Test: Are You Lonely?

W̲e may seek any of countless qualities in a partner, but the ones that truly matter are few in number. The ultimate test of a relationship's health is a simple question: Are you frequently lonely? If you are in a relationship and you say yes, then the relationship is not meeting your most fundamental needs.

"IS THIS HOW I'm supposed to feel," Tonya remembers thinking to herself, "married but alone?"

Tonya's spouse worked long hours at the office, came home, and worked more hours there. When not working, he wanted to dedicate the time to himself. "He would say, 'I need a few minutes here,' which meant don't bother him, don't ask him to do anything or even be there with you.

"I realized that what we had on most days was not that different than if I was a hired hand. I do some things for you, I stay out of your way, I make no demands, I'm grateful for the occasional word of praise."

Tonya gave up on waiting for him to notice the problem. "Subtlety was not getting me much of a response." One day, after a series of long workdays followed by long worknights and a growing feeling of complete invisibility, Tonya moved out. While she went only a few miles away, her point had clearly been made.

Tonya's husband examined his habits, now put in stark relief based on what she'd done. He asked Tonya to forgive him for his thoughtlessness and pledged that he would seek to be her partner in all respects in the future. Two years later, Tonya says, "I feel like I have a true partner now."

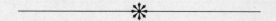

In studies of people in long-term committed relationships, more than a quarter of respondents admitted feeling lonely on a regular basis. Of those, only 8 percent thought their relationship was healthy. (Levine 2000)

17

It's the Little Things That Matter the Most

The peaks of life may be wonderful and the depths of our life painful, but the average day is neither. We define our relationships based not on the best days or the worst days but on the average days. Strive to be supportive in average ways on average days, and you will set in place a major building block of a relationship.

BILL AND KELLY and their five children live on the 250-acre farm where Bill grew up working the land with his father. Bill grows corn and soybeans. He recently took a second job as a crop-insurance adjuster. Kelly works as a manager of a local store.

The stresses of farming were taking a toll on Bill and Kelly. Large bills and a low return for crops would leave Bill sullen one minute, raging the next.

"I'd blow up easy over little things," he said. "Something is out of place, I'm angry about it. Something is not done, I'm angry about it." Like many farmers, Bill resisted the idea of seeking help. He was proud and independent, tough enough to handle his own problems—or so he thought.

"But I looked out my window and wondered, 'What am I going to do to get more land so that I can make a living?' and there weren't any answers. So I just took it out on the people around me.

"I knew I couldn't get these problems solved on my own anymore."

Bill received counseling from a Minnesota state program that began as a means of offering agricultural advice and was later expanded to deal with the great personal stress many farmers were experiencing.

Kelly and Bill both attended counseling sessions through the farmers' program. "There are still trials and tribulations, but nothing like before," Kelly said. Bill said he's learning how to deal more effectively with stress. "I don't get angry like I used to," he said. "I think before I react to things. I put things in perspective."

Interviews with longtime married couples revealed that nine in ten defined their marriage not in relation to the best and worst events of their lives but in relation to typical interactions and typical events. (Appleton and Bohm 2001)

18

A Relationship Requires Two Equals

Imagine two people working on an important project. If the top priority of the project is to complete some specific assignment, you might put one person in charge and assign the two different tasks depending on their abilities. As long as the project is successfully completed, it doesn't matter if one person does a better job or is more committed to the assignment. But what if the top priority of the project is to have the team members like and respect each other? Then putting one person in charge will likely invite feelings of jealousy. And if one person tries harder than the other, feelings of resentment will surely follow. A relationship is, of course, just such a project. Relationships crumble under the weight of imbalance. Neither person can be more important. Neither person can be more involved or committed. Neither person can make all the decisions. Neither person can make all the sacrifices. In the project that is a relationship, no one gets top billing because without two equals there is no relationship.

HE'S AN ATTORNEY. She owns a real estate firm. They value each other, they value the equality of men and women, and they view each other as equals in every respect. But Susan and Trevor, Wisconsin residents who've been married eight years, spent a lot of time arguing about household responsibilities.

Even by Trevor's accounting, Susan handled about 60 percent of the workload from cleaning and shopping to looking after their two children. He was no slouch, they agree, but she did much more, and they argued about it.

"His projects always took precedence," she said. "If I wanted to get something done, I'd also have to pick up the kids, fix some things, and so on."

Then one day Trevor handled a case that put things in perspective. "A business basically had a two-track system for hiring factory workers. Men automatically went into a higher-paying scale that had somewhat more variety in the work. Women automatically went into a lower-paying scale in which their job was exactly the same, every day. On day one, men were given the men's jobs and women the women's jobs, and there was never an opportunity to switch. Never. An individual woman who could do everything and more than a man stayed in the lower-paying, less pleasant job." After taking the case on behalf of a group of women who argued that this system discriminated against them, Trevor couldn't help but reexamine his home life.

"I sat down and was struck—I mean I knew this going in, but I didn't really think about it—but when an emergency strikes, Susan has to handle it. If our daughter gets sick, it's Susan's day that gets sacrificed. If the car needs to go in for service, it's Susan who has to go out of her way. I thought, there's no more justification for automatically making Susan handle this than for assigning those women different jobs automatically."

Trevor's revelation brought a new system in which Susan and Trevor rotate duties that disrupt their days, and Trevor has accepted a number of Susan's least-favorite chores. And in return for Trevor's willingness to adopt a more equal schedule, "We never argue about who is doing what, and we say 'thank you' and 'you're welcome' instead. It is a sacrifice in time and effort, but one that carries rewards tenfold," Susan reports.

The relationships of partners who characterize each other as equal in making decisions, in sacrificing for the relationship, and in performing household chores are likely to last more than twice as long as relationships in which these factors are not equal. (Gilbert and Walker 2001)

19

Beware of Fairy Tales

It may sound ridiculous, but fairy tales matter. Our first conceptions of relationships, love, marriage, and life happily ever after are powerfully influenced by classic stories we read and films we see. While we don't expect anyone to track us down to try magic slippers on our feet, we do expect a certain amount of enchantment to accompany love and life. See the magic of everyday life, of sharing and caring about someone, but don't riddle yourself with expectations of a fairy tale in which the story is strictly about the search for love and the rest of life is just supposed to figure itself out.

"IT'S A WAR against normal people, normal lives, fulfillment, and just about everything else that's good and reasonable," says media critic Sharon Tarver.

Her target? Media depictions of relationships.

"We have one basic model out there. The *Sleepless in Seattle* model, or just about any Meg Ryan movie for that matter, where the perfect person is out there, just waiting to meet you, if only you could find them. Or even worse, *Kate and Leopold,* where her character needs to travel back in time to the 1800s to find someone worthy. The message here is that solid, upstanding citizens all around you need not apply. There's somebody perfect if only you would look.

"And look at the poll results. Ninety-four percent of people in their twenties set their sights on finding their ideal soul mate to marry. Their ideal soul mate! That's going to take some doing.

"What's worse," she adds, "is when you take this model and throw in a little nasty bit of reality—that while we all may be waiting for our perfect soul mate, many of us have entered relationships along the way. Look at something like *The Bridges of Madison County,* where a woman in a loving family drops everything for her perfect man. So what if you marry somebody who's just okay and then meet your true love? Drop him, he wasn't worth it.

"It's chilling, really. The message is 'Don't get married, don't get in a committed relationship—because perfection awaits.' "

Tarver implores people to understand that "Cinderella, Prince Charming, Meg Ryan—these are not real people. Don't get trapped by the sales pitch for them."

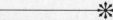

Elements of fairy tales such as Cinderella were present in 78 percent of people's beliefs about romantic love. Those people were more likely to have experienced disillusionment, devastation, and angst in their relationships than were those who gave less credence to fairy tales. (Lockhart 2000)

20

Cultivate a Common Interest

E ach of us wants to be a positive part of our partner's life and have our partner be a positive part of our life. However, much of our day is spent pursuing careers and fulfilling obligations. That's why it is so important that people look for, or develop, common interests in their relationships. Common interests encourage positive communication and fun, and they strengthen the sense of connection between partners.

BERT AND DIANE'S idea of fun is to hop into their canoe and paddle the day away together. The Minnesota couple, married more than three decades, decided to take it a little further, though, and planned a four-month journey through the waters and wilderness on the U.S.-Canada border.

"We both love the boundary waters," said Bert. "It's so incredibly beautiful. The trees, the rocks, and the loons. The smell of the pines. The solitude. And us being together. The beauty is enhanced for us because it takes some effort to get there. We love to paddle in the wilderness."

For their journey there were no time schedules and no deadlines. "We're in no hurry to get back to the pressures of everyday life. The world can go on without us knowing about it," Diane explained.

What do they do with all their time out on the water by day and camping on the water's edge by night? "We talk, or there are times when we don't do a lot of talking, which is fine," said Bert. "We feel like we're each other's best friend, and we're comfortable with each other. I don't think we'll ever get tired of each other."

As for a downside to their common passion? "Mosquitoes. Definitely mosquitoes," he said.

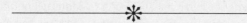

In comparing couples who remained together more than five years with couples who split up, researchers found that the couples who stayed together were 64 percent more likely to be able to identify multiple shared interests. (Bachand and Caron 2001)

21

Treat the Disease, Not the Symptom

Disagreements are inevitable. In trying to address them, many of us adopt a strategy of fixing the immediate problem. If your partner complains that you don't go out and have fun enough, then you try to accommodate the complaint and head out on Saturday night. Generally, though, major complaints present themselves as mere symptoms. That is, the problem isn't what you are doing this Saturday night but a general feeling of boredom that has burdened the relationship. If you address only the immediate symptom, the real problem won't go away.

"IT'S ALMOST too dumb to talk about," Sam admits, but his girlfriend, Laura, was a television vulture. "If you're watching a game, and let's say reading the newspaper at the same time, she'll come in and grab the remote, and the next thing you know, Martha Stewart is on telling us how to make curtains or something.

"I'll say, 'I was watching that,' and she'll say, 'No, you weren't.' And then it's a big thing."

The disagreement kept springing up until Sam and Laura sat down one day to discuss why they were arguing over such matters. Laura said she didn't understand why he got so upset. Sam said he didn't understand why she was lacking in concern for his feelings. Laura said it's just a game on television. But that's not the point, he said.

At a loss for progress, they finally brought in a trusted third party for some help. "My sister said we're both making me-first assumptions—that I was reading and watching the game as if our whole world revolved around me, and that she was snookering the television remote as if I wasn't there. So then we started thinking about ways we could be less selfish around each other, and before long I was avoiding turning on the television unless there was a game I really wanted to see, and she stopped changing the channel when she came into the room. And pretty soon we were looking for ways we could be nice to each other. It is amazing how quickly the petty squabbles go away when you understand the big picture of sharing and caring and really treating each other as you wish to be treated."

Couples who talk to each other about how they disagree, and not just about the disagreement, spend less time arguing. That is, couples who openly share their thoughts and their images related to areas of conflict are 18 percent more likely to report that their disagreements often produce solutions and are 12 percent more likely to say they are satisfied in their relationship. (Palmer-Daley 2001)

22

There's No Point in Putting On a Show

We would expect to find contentment among those who are happy in their relationship and feelings of discontent among people who are unhappy in their relationship. In fact, many people who are discontent are satisfied to remain where they are. They are unhappy with their relationship but have little inclination to end it. Why? They want to remain in their relationship not for the relationship but because they see the social benefits of it. They seek the presentation value to family, friends, and colleagues of being in a relationship. Such a situation is akin to living your life as if it existed for public relations purposes. There is no satisfaction, no fulfillment, no point to being in a relationship that does not meet your needs.

WHEN KELLY RUTHERFORD, an actress who starred on *Melrose Place*, married Carlos Tarajano, a bank executive, the scene was memorable. Rutherford wore a Carolina Herrera gown and toted a three-karat, emerald-encrusted ring on her finger. Guests celebrated in the Sunset Room of the Beverly Hills Hotel late into the night. It was such an event that *InStyle* magazine profiled the spectacular ceremony in its next issue.

By the time the issue hit the newsstands, filled with dazzling pictures of the happy couple, Kelly Rutherford had filed for divorce.

The magazine has also published features on the weddings of comedian Tom Green to actress Drew Barrymore and of actress Courtney

Thorne-Smith to Andrew Conrad after the paperwork had been filed for dissolutions. The marriages of Helen Hunt to Hank Azaria and Jennifer Lopez to Ojani Noa survived past publication date but ended within weeks after they were profiled.

Cognizant of the trend, St. Louis Rams quarterback Kurt Warner, married for five years, declined the chance to be featured in *InStyle*.

David Blankenhorn, a sociologist affiliated with the Institute for American Values in New York, said that this strange pattern is in part a reflection of trends in society as a whole. "When marriage is a show, it's prone to be canceled. We need, as a society, to pay less attention to the appearance of our relationships and more attention to their reality."

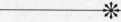

One in five married persons reported that they found their relationship unsatisfying but did not wish to make any changes because of the status value of being married. (Nock 2001)

23

You Make Your Own History

W e've all seen many divorces and countless failed relationships. It is nearly impossible not to take those examples and become somewhat fearful. But the experiences of others aren't always the best guide, just the most obvious one. Take what you can learn from the relationship mistakes and triumphs you witness, but don't limit yourself to reliving someone else's experience.

CHRIS AND ANGEL heard the message all too clearly: "You're too young," their families said again and again. Just out of high school, Chris and Angel were determined to get married anyway.

They had lived just two doors away from each other in Chicago. "I remember the very first thing he ever said to me that made me realize that he was attracted to me," Angel recalls. "He said, 'Oh, that blue dress looks really nice.' But he didn't say that I looked nice in it."

"I was trying to think of something that was acceptable to say," says Chris.

Chris's gentle demeanor and kind heart won her over. They had a lot in common: they shared a desire to help the less fortunate in their community, and both loved running. When Chris proposed, Angel accepted. A few weeks later Angel broke the engagement, worrying that they were rushing things. "I've seen a lot of marriages that didn't work out, and I don't want to go through that," Angel told him.

With differing views on the future of their relationship, the pair soon broke up.

Nevertheless, they continued to see each other on a daily basis—in the hallways, at the office of the magazine where they both worked. Nine months after their breakup, Chris's biggest fear came true. Angel began dating. Angel was convinced, and later Chris agreed, that the path following a broken engagement did not lead back to a relationship.

"There was one point when we decided that we would all be friends," Chris remembers. "At first I thought this was a good, mature idea. I figured it would be healthy and that I could just move on. But, in truth, I couldn't take it. It was too hard for me to see."

But five years of friendship brought a new understanding. "I figured out that I didn't have to give up. I didn't have to say, 'Just because this isn't the way it normally works, I can't do it this way.'" Chris asked Angel out for a date and a few months later asked her to marry him (again). She said yes, and they have been happily married for a decade since.

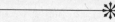

In studies of children of divorced couples, researchers have found no greater tendency to experience divorce or unhappy relationships. Children of divorce are, however, 15 percent more likely to view the strength of their relationship as a mission that requires their sustained effort. (Zink 2000)

24

Maintain Your Sense of Control

In all aspects of your life, you will feel a greater sense of satisfaction and less stress if you maintain a sense of control. You have to recognize that your decisions shape your life, regardless of what else might be happening around you. A healthy relationship will foster this sense that your decisions matter, while an unhealthy relationship will make you feel your decisions are irrelevant. Seek to maintain your sense of control in everything you do.

MADGE AND EDDIE have been married for more than seven decades. During their marriage they've seen the world change and twelve presidents come and go.

What put so much staying power in their wedding vows? "Love," said Madge. "That's all."

There was, of course, mutual respect and patience. And what Madge calls "a Midwestern mind-set, a sort of stick-to-itiveness common among folks from a certain time."

Eddie says their arguments helped a lot, too—little disagreements, each followed quickly by forgiveness. "Say something didn't go just right. We'd get mad. We might not speak to each other. But later that day, you wouldn't know it," said Eddie.

"Well," Madge added, "he might pout for a while."

For Madge, such marital know-how came from "good old common sense. You have to give and take. But you've got to keep control of yourself all the time. Never take it too far.

"Anyone who says they never argue, they are either dad-blum liars or they don't give a hoot," she said.

If things were too much for Madge she took an occasional weekend for herself. "I still like to be alone sometimes," she said. "If you can't stand yourself, how can you stand anybody else?"

But, as Madge is quick to point out, "I'm still in love. I love the old bugger and wouldn't want to get rid of him."

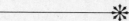

People with a sense of control in their lives, in both career and relationship, were 66 percent more likely to report feeling happy and satisfied. (Chou and Chi 2001)

25

Money Can't Buy Love, but It Can Buy Stress

What is the single most important part of your life? It's not money. It never has been, and it never will be. But how many times has a disagreement about money—how to spend it, how to get it, how much is enough—gotten in the way of your enjoying time with loved ones? When we let the superficial things get in the way of the substantial, our relationships cannot possibly remain healthy. We will be disturbed if we don't have enough money and even disappointed when we do have enough money because it will not bring us the joy and fulfillment we need. Put money in its place—behind what really matters to you.

"THE AVERAGE PERSON abuses money," says Steve Rhode of Myvesta, a financial counseling program headquartered in Maryland. He means that addictive tendencies can show up in how we use money as well as how we use substances. At Myvesta Rhode counsels people on smart money use, and he also runs a program addressing life and relationship skills because he sees them as nearly inseparable from money use.

"Money abuse is the inability to control ourselves with regard to spending," Rhode says. "It is a recurrent, often unconscious, use of money to overcome underlying issues. Our society recognizes that people abuse alcohol, drugs, and food and that they need help to overcome those issues, but what about people who abuse money?"

Rhode warns that what makes our use of money even more dangerous is that it is often overlooked, treated as a frivolous situation instead
of as a problem. "Many people assume that it's normal to be unable to
control their money. It's not. People get stuck because they deny that a
problem exists. Denial holds them back from finding a path to peace of
mind and conquering their money issues."

He continues, "People conceal their money habits, argue over money
habits, let money habits dictate who they are. There is just no way to
deny that your money habits will affect your relationship. But a commitment to healthy money habits means a help to your relationship."

Rhode's message to clients is to focus on what is truly important to
them while monitoring their spending impulses. "Spending money is a
surface solution to a core problem. We try to fill up holes by spending
money on them. There's no point trying to fill the holes in your life with
money because you can keep pouring cash in them and you will never
fill them."

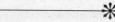

Financial disagreements are a significant source of conflict in more than
half of all relationships. Interestingly, this problem occurs regardless of
income level. (Goldscheider 1999)

26

There Are No Mind Readers

You want support and comfort because of a trying situation. You want your partner to understand the situation and the difficulty you face and make you feel better—even if you don't actually say these things or explain the situation or make sure your partner fully understands what is going on. We often set up our partners to fail us in these situations by not fully disclosing our feelings and the situation as we perceive it. When you need support, explain the situation. The response you receive will be not only more meaningful but also more powerful.

ED WORKS in a California-based public relations firm. His boss is his wife, Gwen.

"For spousal business relationships to work, it takes mutual admiration of business skills and total honesty," Ed says. "I have a lot of respect for Gwen and her abilities. If she were less proficient, I probably wouldn't have come to work for her.

"You have to be pretty secure in your masculinity, though," he admits. "But Gwen is a genius, and I think I'm good at what I do."

Gwen also admires her husband's skills. "He could sell ice to Eskimos," she says.

Ed thinks that this setup would have been impossible a generation ago. "My father would not be able to do this, but I have no problem whatsoever with women being in charge," Ed said. "It's working without ego, based on competencies, not gender."

Despite all their mutual respect, problems inevitably arise. "Ed will get so wrapped up in making sure everything runs right that he will turn and give me a direction like he's talking to an employee," Gwen said. "That irritates me."

But Gwen doesn't hide that irritation from Ed. Neither does Ed shy away from noting when he feels Gwen is bringing her office role home. Gwen admitted, "It's difficult to be in charge in a business sense, then not carry that home. Ed's the only one who can rein me in."

Such circumstances are inevitable and highlight the need for open communication to head off conflicts. "We have to say what we mean—with no underlying messages," said Ed. "If the emotional message is different from the content, that's a problem."

"We don't hide things," agreed Gwen. "Being forthright is the key."

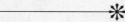

Researchers found that those who are more direct in seeking support from their partner are 61 percent more likely to feel they received the support they wanted than are those who avoid explaining their needs. (Fitness 2001)

27

There's No Need to Hurry

The age at which people choose to marry has been rising every decade for the past hundred years. The age at which those who have children first do so has also been rising every decade for the past hundred years. People are starting these life-altering courses later and later for many reasons, including financial pressures and a desire to obtain and maintain independence. There's no need to hurry. Relationships are not a race, and there's no prize for finishing first.

MOVIE STUDIO CHIEF Barry Diller and fashion designer Diane von Furstenberg had been in each other's lives, either as friends or as a couple, for more than twenty-five years.

"He said it first," von Furstenberg recalled. "He said, 'Wouldn't it be nice?' We always say we're going to do it, maybe Christmas, maybe my birthday, and we don't." And with that, the longtime friends decided to get married.

Off they marched on Diller's fifty-ninth birthday to City Hall in New York for a civil ceremony. They had to squeeze through reporters and photographers who were tipped off to the event by friends. "There was no serious planning," von Furstenberg said, "and that's the way I like it."

She continues, "We've been together for so long, it's like we already are married. Whatever happens, though, nothing will change. We love each other. Our relationship has always been based on truth and a trust between us. After all these years, this feels very natural."

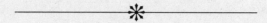

Marrying later in life has no negative effect on satisfaction with the relationship or with life. (Juang and Silbereisen 2001)

28

Friends Speak from Experience—Their Own

When we want validation for our decisions we often turn to friends for advice and approval. But our friends can speak only from their own experience. And while in most things the words of an experienced veteran would be highly valued, in making decisions about your relationship, your friends will be speaking from their experience, not yours. Neither you nor your situation is something that your friends have experience with. Value their friendship, but understand that their advice applies primarily to themselves.

JAMES AND RENEE of Georgia owe their entire relationship to mutual friends, a married couple who brought them together on a group date.

They didn't immediately hit it off. "I had never met anyone so arrogant," says Renee.

"I thought she needed a lot of work," James remembers.

Nevertheless, their friends clandestinely brought them together a second time. Things went a little better. They began a relationship, and three years later they married.

Their marriage began with some bumps that James attributes to advice he received from one of the friends who fixed him up with Renee. "He's married, and he had a lot to say about what to expect in a marriage—things you shouldn't allow to change in your life just because you're getting married. He basically said that if you do things right when you first get married, then you'll have a lifetime of reward. If you do things wrong—if you don't lay down the right expectations—you'll be paying for that for a lifetime."

James implemented the advice, making it clear to Renee what things he did not intend to sacrifice for marriage. The advice, James now admits, "was a disaster." James and Renee argued all the time, and instead of setting himself up for a lifetime of reward, James was setting himself up for a quick divorce.

He soon decided to throw out the advice. "I realized pretty early on that to stay together, each partner must make the other number one. I realized that I could love someone as much as I love myself—and even more. And that the reward is in the caring, not in the selfishness."

When asked to comment on a young person starting out in a relationship, 92 percent of participants drew from their own personal experience to make conclusions and offer advice. (Protinsky and Coward 2001)

29

Drink Less

Excessive alcohol consumption poses many dangers to physical health. But it also threatens the stability of relationships. Long-term sustained drinking patterns affect emotional states and views of the world, which means that light drinkers are happier and more confident in their relationships.

ALTHOUGH ACTING is the family business, Stephen Baldwin has had to struggle against comparing himself to his older and more famous brothers Alec, Daniel, and William. While trying to make a name for himself, he has pursued many parts that portray characters on the outside looking in. "These characters have a feeling of emptiness from everything they carry around. They exude a detachment, which they use as a shield. It's a feeling they've had to create for themselves after being exposed to the worst elements of this world."

Emptiness has been all too easy to tap into for Baldwin. He attributes a series of failed relationships to the problems with alcohol he experienced in the early years of his acting career. He turned his life around a decade ago. "It feels great," he says. "I'm no longer harming myself, which means I can be there for someone else."

That someone else is his wife, Kennya Deodata. Baldwin says, "The smartest thing I ever did was marry Kennya."

He adds, "There are two very important words that husbands have to learn. They are *Yes, dear*. We had a home near Tucson, because we liked the area when I was shooting *The Young Riders*. Then Kennya decided we should live in upstate New York. Hey, that's fine." He will do what it takes to promote happiness in his marriage because "marriage and fatherhood are the only true realities that I experience. I'm in this kooky business that is not rooted in reality."

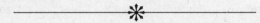

Over the course of a decade, a low frequency of alcohol consumption was associated with a 57 percent greater chance of maintaining a happy long-term relationship than was moderate to heavy drinking. (Prescott and Kendler 2001)

30

Decide Whether You Want to Win or Be Happy

Everyone argues—of course. Disagreements are an inevitable part of two people trying to coexist. But at their root, arguments pose only one real question: Do you want to win by showing how right you are, or do you want to compassionately come to a resolution with your partner? You can win all the arguments you want and feel good about always being right. But you will not have helped yourself in the slightest. Or you can give up thinking about who won and lost because, in truth, either you both win the argument or you both lose.

COLMAN MCCARTHY teaches conflict resolution to children, adults, and couples. He tells people to approach conflict in a healthy way.

First, he says, "define the situation objectively. What is the situation, and what needs to happen to improve it? This simple step is crucial. Sociologists report that in as many as 75 percent of husband-wife fights, the combatants are battling over different issues. The husband may be enraged over what his wife said or did that morning. The wife is out of control over what her husband said or did ten weeks ago. They can't settle their conflict because they don't know what it's about."

The next step, McCarthy says, is to "realize the contest involved. It's not you against me, it's you and me against the problem. Most people— and nations for that matter—go into battle convinced, 'I'm right, you're wrong; I'm good, you're evil.' Even if one side does win, the first reaction of the loser is, 'I want a rematch. I'll come back with meaner words, harder fists, and bigger bombs. Then you'll learn, then you'll be good, and then we'll have peace forever.' This is an illusion, but few can give it up." Focus not on the other person, he says, but on the problem that stands between you. "By focusing on the problem, and not the person with the problem, a climate of cooperation instead of competition can be enhanced."

He continues, "Then start with what's doable. Restoration of peace can't be done quickly. If it took a long time for the dispute to begin, it will take time to end it. Almost always, it's a laughably small wound that causes the first hurt in a relationship. But then, ignoring the smallness takes on a size of its own. Ignoring the problem becomes larger than the original problem."

McCarthy admits that sometimes the partners in conflict are so emotionally wounded that nothing can help. "But large numbers of conflicts can be resolved, provided the strategies for peacemaking are known. Gandhi said, 'Don't bring your opponents to their knees, bring them to their senses.'"

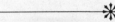

People who maintain a compassionate spirit during disagreements with their partner, considering not just the virtue of their position but the virtue of their partner, have 34 percent fewer disagreements, and the disagreements last 59 percent less time. (Wu 2001)

31

A Sense of Humor Helps

A good joke can brighten any day, bringing joy to both the teller and the listener. In a relationship, a good sense of humor helps to make the average day more fun, and it lessens the burden of the bad days. This humor must be directed toward positive directions, of course. Negative, biting jokes only serve to heighten tensions.

VIVA AND JERRY of Minneapolis have been hosting *Viva and Jerry's Country Videos* on local cable access for more than a decade. They are the Sonny and Cher of no-budget, Minneapolis-area cable television. Their show is a confounding mix of bad puns, filched country music, and product spoofs, and it has drawn something of a cult following.

Viewers are attracted to the kitsch and clatter of the show, to the silly spoofs on products pulled out of discount store bins and bought at garage sales. But most of all, they are lured by Viva and Jerry. The playful banter and constant fawning these two do over each other convey an uncommon television image: a couple in their sixties who are really in love.

Both Viva and Jerry enjoy a good joke—actually, they also enjoy bad ones. Viva told viewers why she went out with Jerry in the first place: "This is the first guy that gave me goose bumps," she says. Then she holds up two plastic geese with little bumps on them. "Here they are."

"Yah," says Jerry, giving his trademark thumbs-up sign.

In between the laughs, Viva dispenses her own philosophy of life. "So I tell people, never give up on love; it took me forty-five years to luck out."

Though they appear gleefully happy on the show, the two admit their relationship isn't perfect. They argue, as do all couples. "It's hard work," Viva says of marriage. "You have to learn to live with quirks. Jerry, he leaves toothpicks all around."

But the complaints are few. "You look cuter than a monkey," says Viva.

"Don't go ape over me, hey," Jerry says.

After twelve years together, they very much enjoy each other's company. The show is part of what keeps them going, something odd and funny—and, in a strange way, meaningful—to share. Couples need that, Viva says. Which is why they spend half of their free day putting on a show that pays them nothing.

"It gives us something to look forward to," said Viva. "And it's given us new horizons. At our age, we're still meeting all these new people and doing things we would have never done. And all with a laugh."

When both partners in a relationship thought the other had a good sense of humor, 67 percent less conflict was reported than in couples where neither thought the other had a good sense of humor. (De Koning and Weiss 2002)

32

Think Beyond the Engagement

A friend announces her engagement, and feelings of envy soon can overwhelm us. She appears the picture of happiness and contentment, a person with a relationship and a plan for the rest of her life. In the face of this example, many will ask why they are not in a relationship, not married, or not nearly as happy. But the engagement period is an unrealistic point of comparison. Those who are engaged are flush with the excitement of a newly made major decision, which, whether good or bad, will fill them with anticipation. The nervous energy of the first day of school and the excitement of buying a house are also emotions born of a unique time. Living in the house, going to school, and being married are entirely different matters from the buildup that precedes them. Don't judge your own life by comparing it to unique moments that are not meant to be sustained.

VERMONT NATIVES Doug and Gloria looked forward to their marriage, and their engagement was a dream come true for both.

Even after the divorce that followed four years later, Gloria admits they have a lot in common. "I think our qualities complement each other in many ways, but we were, and are, incompatible. There were too many points of contention."

Gloria cautions that the "pictures in your head of the perfect house with the white picket fence and the glamorous life can overwhelm all logic" when engagements occur. She says, "Now I view marriage as more of a work in progress and less a fantasy."

Indeed, as a freelance writer, Gloria has pondered that idea in her essays. "I'm interested in the unhealthy extremes we all too often live between," she says. "Engagement is no more a fairy tale than divorce is a prison sentence. Neither my ex-husband nor I became anarchists with green hair or anything like that after the divorce. We've lived full lives and happy lives, but not magical lives."

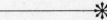

Psychologists find that "idealistic distortion," the tendency to make unrealistically positive assessments of our relationship and our partner, is more than twice as great during an engagement period as during the dating that precedes it or the marriage that follows it. (Bonds-Raacke, Bearden, Carriere, Anderson, and Nicks 2001)

33

See the Friendship in Your Relationship

The two closest relationships in your life are likely to be between you and a partner and between you and a best friend. But for many, feelings of closeness, supportiveness, affection, and good communication are stronger with a best friend. This imbalance can be a source of frustration and disappointment in your relationship. Of course, your friendship has an advantage over your relationship; the great struggles, dilemmas, and debates in your life are likely to happen within your relationship, and by comparison your friendship looks easier or better. But if you see the friendship in your relationship, you can recognize that the difficulties of a relationship are a prelude to their strength.

KEITH AND LENA did things backward. First they moved in together, and then they fell in love.

They were both part-time students with full-time jobs when they met in an early childhood education class. He was looking for a room; she was looking for a roommate to share an apartment. Ten months of sharing a home brought them very close to each other.

"Our entire relationship was based on friendship," said Lena. "I was dating someone else; he was going on dates." But they shared much in common, including budding careers in education.

Then came the summer.

Keith took a job with a camp in Michigan but found himself on the phone every day with Lena. She would call for little things, like what to do with his mail. The apartment was empty without him, she said.

Keith's codirector at the camp put the bug in his ear. "She kept telling me, 'You're in love,'" Keith said.

Soon after, Lena broke off her relationship with her boyfriend. "Being with Keith made me realize how nice a guy could be," she said.

When Keith returned in August and walked up the stairs to their third-floor apartment, he realized how thrilled he was to see her.

They shared their first kiss. "That's when I knew," Keith said. "But we already lived together. We had to figure out how to start dating someone we'd already seen in their underwear first thing in the morning."

The couple credit their happy marriage to the friendship they built first. "We got to know each other" before dating, Keith said. "We knew everything already. There was none of that posturing."

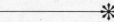

For three out of five people, best friends were thought to be more support-ive, more open in communication, and the source of stronger feelings of affection than relationship partners. (Vinograde 2001)

34

The Most Time Is Not the Best Time

If we have found the one person in the world we most want to spend our time with, then why not spend as much time together as possible? Because relationships thrive on the quality, not the quantity, of contact. For most people, a little distance every day is necessary for their own independent interests and needs. Time apart also serves to strengthen the relationship by giving both partners a chance to feel an active need for each other and to experience the pleasure of reuniting.

CARLA AND BRIAN run a bus line that provides tours around Boston. They divorced after a fifteen-year marriage but continue to amicably operate the business they started together ten years ago.

Carla says the pressures of growing a business together put stresses on their relationship. "When we decided to end the marriage, we did it with a small realization that we had perhaps put more into the business than we had into our marriage," Carla said. "We made a sad but conscious decision to save the business and let the marriage go."

She emphasizes the need for couples who work together especially to have a firm foundation in open communication and conflict resolution, since they'll be spending all day, every day, in each other's company. She thinks difficulty in those areas was at least partially responsible for the breakup of her marriage.

Brian agrees. "We all have a tendency when we're under stress and things are not going so well to blame others. It's a particular risk for couples who are in business together. If they're facing business problems or personal challenges in the business, it's just really easy to turn on your spouse and blame each other." He advises couples who work together to develop significant independent activities away from work—and from each other. "What happens for a lot of couples in business is they end up being in each other's space so intensely that between home and work, they can really start to lose perspective."

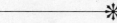

Seventy-six percent of newly retired married couples say they face a challenge dealing with the greatly increased time spent in each other's company. (Szinovacz and Schaffer 2000)

35

Reduce TV Time

Television introduces us to some unrealistically positive images of relationships and many unrealistically negative images as well. Television contributes to several problems and few, if any, solutions for our relationship situation. Take the time you would otherwise spend on television, and put it to use on your relationship instead.

FRANK VESPE is the executive director of the TV-Turnoff Network based in Washington, D.C. He cites some alarming statistics. "The time per day the TV is on in the average U.S. home is seven hours, forty minutes. More Americans have televisions than indoor plumbing. Almost half of all Americans admit they watch too much TV."

While the quantity of television consumption is disturbing, Vespe is even more troubled by the implications. "Watching TV is an isolating experience," he said. "It's bad for our bodies, it's bad for our brains. The neocortex, or part of the brain that deals with personal relationships, evolves through interaction—and TV requires zero interaction. It saps our family time. Many of us spend more time with the tube than with our families. It draws you in. It's a bad habit."

Vespe's group runs an annual campaign encouraging people to give up all television for a week. "For most people, just seeing that their world will continue without television—in fact, their life will be better without television—is really an eye opener. Because one of the most insidious aspects of our television use is that for most of us it is automatic. The television is there, so we turn it on. There's something on so we watch it. If we did anything else so randomly and thoughtlessly we'd look crazy, but when we thoughtlessly use the television, no one questions us."

Margaret and Bob heard about Vespe's efforts and decided to give up their televisions for a week. "I feel like I don't really want to watch, then I do anyway. It's the same reaction you have as at a car wreck. You look even if you know you shouldn't," Margaret said. Margaret thinks her TV-free week had dramatic effects. "We had fallen into a routine. We wanted to get back to some family time. It's so easy to sit there and glaze over. But, we made it for a week—now we'll see if we can keep it off. This will be a good test for us."

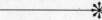

People who watched an above-average amount of television per day were 26 percent less likely to be satisfied with their relationship status than were people who watched a below-average amount of television per day. (Hetsroni 2000)

36

The World Will Intrude
on Your Relationship

It's easy to say that our partner is not responsible for our view of the world, yet when life gets rough, many of us turn a more jaundiced eye toward our relationship. The fact of the matter is that events outside your relationship will color your assessment of your personal life. If you feel negative about other aspects of your life, this will affect your evaluation of your relationship and your feelings toward your partner. Recognize this tendency, and remember that improving your relationship may involve changing things that don't directly involve your partner.

JOHN AND SARAH have the kind of relationship people take note of. "Our love is like a love song," said Sarah, who confesses to being a hopeless romantic. "It's a committed and caring love that grows deeper and deeper day by day."

They didn't develop a resilient relationship by magic. It took respect, sharing their feelings, empathy, and a lot of laughter to keep their relationship exciting over more than twenty-five years.

Their love and commitment were almost lost in the face of a tragic event. In 1997 their only daughter was killed in an accident. The grief was overwhelming. Neither John nor Sarah could function. Home didn't feel like home. They didn't seem to be themselves. Their marriage was nothing more than a numbness that pervaded their days.

There were no easy answers. There were no answers at all. So they took to blaming the only targets that were available, each other. "It wasn't rational, but we saw all kinds of ways to deflect our true feelings about what happened and make this harder on each other," John said.

Even as their individual pain was so great that they had little left to offer each other, they both realized that though they could never be the same, they would both have to fight to keep their relationship from being another victim of the accident. Sarah explained, "We knew, even though our hearts were broken, they were empty, that the bond between us could live on if we let it. We wept and wept, but soon we wept with each other. And while we will always have pain, our dedication to each other helped us out of that valley in our life."

People who had a sense of optimism about the future and maintained a positive outlook on the world were 42 percent more likely to evaluate their relationship positively than were people who had negative feelings about the rest of their life and the outside world. (Symmonds-Mueth 2000)

37

Gentlemen Prefer the Same Things Ladies Prefer

We have stereotypes about the things men want in a woman and the things women want in a man. These are the kinds of things we sometimes joke about. But at the same time, many of us believe them to be true, and we try to adapt ourselves to fit the model of what we think potential partners are looking for. The truth of the matter is that men and women today are looking for the same things. The stereotypes may have been true at one time, but today it's more likely that the things you are looking for are the same things your potential partner is looking for.

WHEN PSYCHOLOGISTS WANT to have a better idea of what men and women are looking for in a potential mate, they turn to the personals—not to find a date, but to read about how people describe themselves and describe their desired mate.

Psychologist Thomas Cash has analyzed thousands of ads. "People reveal themselves in these ads in a way that is really unique. They define who they are succinctly, perhaps overly optimistically, and they define the essence of what they are looking for—sometimes suggesting great depth, and oftentimes suggesting a most superficial level of their thinking."

Traditionally, researchers such as Professor Cash expected to find great differences between what men and women wanted. But Cash's recent studies reveal that women are just as likely as men to make requests regarding appearance or background when describing the desired soul mate. "In other words, as women gain economic power, women can be just as frivolous as men and look for a cute butt," says Cash.

"The age-old, evolutionary contract between men and women, in which men provided security and women comfort, is changing. Men and women are now looking for the same thing."

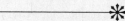

Long-term studies of partner preferences, conducted over a sixty-year period, find that men and women were once quite distinct in their ideas about an ideal mate. Today, however, the core desires of men and women are nearly identical. (Buss, Shackelford, Kirkpatrick, and Larsen 2001)

38

Love Is Blind but Life Isn't Always

Expectations about who you are allowed to marry are slowly vanishing. For example, society has evolved past the point of expecting people to marry only others of the same race or ethnicity. Yet even while there is no reason for you to exclude groups of people as potential partners, you must recognize the challenges you will face and embrace them. Some people are still likely to see any departure from their expectations and traditions as a threat to themselves. Cross-cultural relationships can be burdened with the strain of dealing with the world or fortified by a mutual response to close-mindedness.

WHEN ANNA and her boyfriend, Leroy, decided to get married, they had to leave their native Colorado for the ceremony. The year was 1953, and the state of Colorado did not allow interracial marriages. Although Anna and Leroy headed for New Mexico for the wedding, they returned to Colorado for their life.

They made a happy life together and had five children. But when they were out together in public, Anna and Leroy were regularly subjected to disapproval, ranging from scornful looks to racial slurs. Although Anna and Leroy felt the ugliness of racism, they were also blessed with the intelligence and fortitude to overcome it.

Anna was never one to flinch in the face of racism. In the 1960s she became the local chairperson of the Congress of Racial Equality, staffing picket lines in front of stores that practiced discriminatory hiring policies and facing down epithets hurled loud and clear at the band of protesters. When the infamous Bull Connor, the Birmingham, Alabama, police commissioner who epitomized racial intolerance, was invited to speak in Denver, Anna showed up to lead the picketing of his appearance.

Even today, Anna admits, "There's always that potential for the unexpected when people see Leroy and me. You like to think people won't be ugly anymore, but they are." But she prefers not to dwell on painful moments such as that. In fact, "I've tried to forget about all that because it was so awful." Instead, she focuses on sweeter moments. "Our life together has not been easy, but it has been wonderful. And while progress is slower than we would like, there has been progress. We feel a greater sense of community today—that sense of belonging that happens when we connect to each other as human beings."

Interracial couples who feel empowered by their commitment to each other are three times as likely to remain partners after a year as are interracial couples who feel like their relationship makes them outsiders. (McFadden 2001)

39

Balance Depends on
Which Way You Lean

W e all know that we should strive to balance our lives. We need
to do things in moderation. But what you should do to improve
differs depending on which direction you naturally head in. For those
who work long hours and focus much of their attention on their career,
greater commitment to their relationship and family time must become
a priority. But for those whose focus is the family, greater time working
outside the home actually increases the health of relationships and family life.

HE WRITES, directs, helps run a theater company he's a founding member
of, and in his spare time stars as Ross in the television hit *Friends*. But
David Schwimmer also recognizes the limits of his work. "I find it sad
that everyone wants their fifteen minutes of fame and we are so con-
sumed by it. It has never been comfortable to me. I don't hang with a
lot of celebrities. And I don't go to Hollywood parties. I hear about these
parties at big directors' and stars' and producers' homes, and I guess I'm
not really interested."

Schwimmer says one thing he has in common with his character,
Ross, is their depth. "Not everything is frivolous to Ross; there's a seri-
ousness about him in terms of how he thinks about relationships, the
family."

Nonetheless, Schwimmer says there is a void in his life where a relationship and family belong. "I'm a workaholic, and that has gotten in the way. I have not been able to find a healthy balance between my work life and my personal life. It's a flaw in my character, and I can't seem to find the balance yet." He hopes that balance may come when *Friends* has finished its course. "Maybe it's as simple as waiting for the show to end and moving back to Chicago. That time will come, and my life will change."

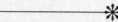

Studies find that the balance between work life and personal life is consistently different for men and women. Most women express more satisfaction with their family as they work more hours outside of the home. Most men express less satisfaction with their family life as they work more hours outside of the home. (Marks, Huston, Johnson, and MacDermid 2001)

40

A Relationship by Any Other Name Is Just as Important

There are marriages that last forever and marriages that last for days. There are people living together for a lifetime, and people living together for hours. What your relationship is called is not what will determine how long it lasts. Decisions about how you spend your life and who you spend it with are just as important whether or not it's called a marriage. Your need to remain committed and supportive every day is just as necessary whether or not you are married. A relationship is what two people make of it, and it will prosper as long as those two people can make it last—regardless of what we call it.

PETE AND VANESSA do not feel inclined to declare their love in front of some anonymous official in a municipal building or in a church. So they have never married—not when they moved in together, not when they bought their first house, not when they had their son, now sixteen.

"We said that if our child were to be harassed at school, we'd think of doing it," said Pete, who has lived with Vanessa for twenty-three years. "But it was never an issue."

Vanessa admits that their decision has been the source of some awkwardness, "My mom has probably lied to some of her friends—well, not lied, but not told the complete truth." But she thinks there is a more important truth. "Love and marriage—they often go together, but it is certainly possible to have one without the other—a marriage with very little commitment or a very committed unmarried couple," she says.

Pete says the questions of when and whether to marry are increasingly seen as deeply personal choices free from the traditional moral judgments of community, family, or church. "The most important thing, it seems to me, is the quality of the relationship between the members of the couple, not whether or not they are married."

While 63 percent of couples who live together think marriage would significantly change their relationship, levels of commitment, supportiveness, and sharing once exclusively seen among married people are now just as common among those living together. (Bumpass and Sweet 2001)

41

The Future Matters More Than the Past

When a relationship has a successful history, some may imagine that the work has already been accomplished. But that is no more true than imagining that successful gardeners can skip watering and fertilizing this year because of their good track record. The fact that you have experience and confidence in your relationship means that you know what needs to be done. It does not mean that you can ignore things that need to be done because you've done them before. The task of a successful relationship never ends because the point of a relationship is to build toward the future, not the past.

SEVENTY VALENTINE'S DAYS have passed since Meyer and Nellie met. And sixty-eight of them since they married. But that didn't stop Meyer from navigating the streets outside their New York City retirement center to buy his wife a box of chocolates this past February 14.

"We've never stopped caring for each other," Nellie explains with pride. "He's always been my guardian."

A formal dinner was held recently at their retirement center to honor Meyer and Nellie for being the longest-married couple in New York City.

In fact, their relationship began when Herbert Hoover was president and the country was in the throes of the Great Depression. "We weren't thinking of depressions then," Nellie says. "We had other things in mind."

Despite their rich past together, Nellie thinks their relationship has prospered in the here and now. "It's as simple as this," Nellie says: "we love each other!"

After sitting in the retirement home's reception room during the afternoon, posing for photographers on hand to mark the occasion, the couple decided to return to their apartment to rest up for their big night. "Come on, kiddo," said Meyer playfully before helping her up, "let's go upstairs."

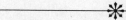

Satisfaction in a relationship is eight times more reliant on recent feelings and the ability to perceive improvements than it is based on the history of the relationship. (Karney and Frye 2002)

42

You Don't Have to See Eye to Eye on Everything

What we see in the world is not a pure, objective view of reality but a perspective on reality based in part on our predispositions. Some have argued that the key to successful communication in a relationship is taking advantage of this process by finding someone who looks at things the same way you do. In other words, find someone who sees the world the same way you do, and you will find someone who will see a relationship the same way you do. Despite the logic behind the theory, in reality, relationship success does not depend on seeing things the same way. Instead, respect for the other person's perspective is far more important than constant agreement with it.

WHEN PSYCHOLOGISTS asked longtime married couples what was missing from their wedding vows, many of them talked about understanding and respecting differences.

"I vow to understand and accept the fact that it is okay to agree to disagree," suggested Mary, a study participant. "It took me a long time to realize, 'Oh, we don't have to agree on everything.'" It really bothered her when she couldn't make her husband completely agree on something that mattered to her. Now, after two decades of marriage, "it saves time and creates a better relationship when neither one of us has to try to change the other person.

"I think about it this way: Who is exactly like you? Who agrees with absolutely everything you think? You. Just you. That's it. But you are not married to yourself; you are married to another person. And for every idea of yours that you want appreciated, respected, or at least tolerated, there are ideas of your spouse you will have to put up with."

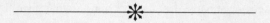

The number of areas couples disagree about does not predict how much time they spend arguing. That is, couples who shared many common opinions were no more likely to positively rate their communication habits or relationship overall than were people who had fewer opinions in common. (Dufore 2000)

43

Be Open with Each Other

It might surprise you to learn that you cannot tell whether a relationship is happy or unhappy just by knowing whether good things or bad things are happening to a couple. But think about it. Many people in strong and vital relationships are suffering through some kind of difficulty in life, while people who seem to have everything one could ever want are in crumbling relationships. The difference is not the circumstances; the difference is how the partners connect with each other. People in healthy relationships share what they are going through, good or bad, with their partners.

Don't hold back—anything. In sharing your reality, you will be sharing your life, and the bond you make in the process will help you through anything.

RAOUL FELDER has a unique perspective on relationships. He's a happily married divorce attorney.

"I don't believe you have to be happy in what you're doing," he said. "That's a myth. I hate what I do—representing people in the most acrimonious, bitter divorces." Felder spends his days representing celebrity clients as they dissolve their marriages and seek an equitable share of their marital assets. He's represented one of Johnny Carson's wives, one of Elizabeth Taylor's husbands, and Mike Tyson's first ex-wife.

How does Raoul Felder manage the task of being a top attorney and a dedicated family man? "In both my marriage and my career, I succeed because I am open. I am open with my wife and open with my clients." Felder stresses the benefits of full, clear communication. "A good lawyer has to be able to write, read, and speak with total clarity, and that's very rare today," he said. "A good husband needs to do the same, to share everything, to include your spouse in your day, your life, your thoughts." Lawyers get in trouble with their client or partners with each other when "they don't know where each other is going, or where they went. I practice the opposite of that."

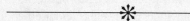

In studies of marriages of various lengths, couples with a high degree of intimacy between the husband and wife—that is, couples who shared their innermost thoughts—were 62 percent more likely to describe their marriage as happy. (Pallen 2001)

44

Accentuate the Positive in All Aspects of Your Life

Logically, our feelings toward our relationship, our job, our family, and our friends should be independent of one another. A good day at work shouldn't make our relationship better, and a bad day at work shouldn't make our relationship less happy. Logic does not always rule our feelings, though. In truth, we tend to allow our feelings about one major aspect of our lives to affect our feelings about other, unrelated, aspects of our lives. Dwelling on the negative side of part of your life will encourage you to dwell on the negative side of your relationship. Avoiding the negative and emphasizing the positive aspects of your life will encourage you to see positives in your relationship.

HIS NAME IS Jason. He's twenty-six and smart. He's good-looking. He's a software programmer, finishing up his master's degree in engineering. He loves music and movies, and he's very well read. He's churchgoing, family oriented, thoughtful.

And he hasn't been out on a date in quite some time. He's pretty sure it has something to do with the wheelchair he's in.

Many disabled people say they've battled issues like these since adolescence. Their desire for romance and family is no different from anyone else's, yet their opportunities for those experiences are much more limited than they are for people without disabilities.

"It's hard to get people to think of you in a dating light," Jason said. "There is a tendency in our society to put people in boxes, and if you have a disability, the disability becomes the defining attribute. I'm a professional, I'm intelligent, I'm a brother and a son, and I'm a human being who happens to have some coordination issues from an injury. To me, this is just part of being Jason."

A friend of Jason's who also has a disability gave him this advice: Live your life, feel good about who you are, but don't be too optimistic about dating. You need to be realistic about how most people feel and recognize that they think dating a disabled person is too much work.

"I understood what he was trying to say, but that's a terribly negative view, and I'm not at that point yet," said Jason. "I envision myself being married and having a family."

When asked to discuss disappointments, frustrations, and other negative aspects of their lives, people were 28 percent more likely to say something negative about their relationship than they were when first asked about positive aspects of their lives. (Caughlin and Huston 2002)

45

It Helps to Be Friends

Imagine you were going to take a long car ride with someone. A really long ride. Days. Weeks. Years. Decades. All this time spent in close proximity to one other person. You would want that person to be a friend. What would sustain that contact would not be momentary glimpses of excitement or delight but rather friendship, a mutual feeling of respect, admiration, and interest. Long-term relationships survive and thrive on a long-term foundation of friendship.

CALIFORNIANS MATT and Claire have been friends for forty years. They've been married for five.

They met in grade school and shared their first kiss a few years later when they attended the same summer camp. In high school a game of spin the bottle gave them an opportunity for a second kiss. They were averaging about a kiss every five years. "Things were a lot tamer in those days," Claire says with a laugh.

While their relationship did not blossom into something more serious, they remained friends over the years. Though they lived in different states and were busy with their lives, they renewed their acquaintance every five years at their high school reunion. At the reunions Matt, as master of ceremonies, always grabbed the microphone to announce, "I see my old flame is present, and I'm still in love with her." They talked of old times and new times, discussed their lives and families, and offered support to each other. And they always shared a special dance.

At their thirtieth reunion, both Matt and Claire were newly single. They sat together. They danced. They talked and talked. And laughed.

They made plans. After the reunion, Matt flew out to see Claire several times. A year later, more than forty years after their first kiss, they were married.

They both see their love as inseparable from their friendship. "She's my best friend, and I'm hers," Matt says.

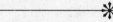

In studies of people happily married more than three decades, the quality of friendship between the partners was the single most frequently cited factor in the relationships' success. (Bachand and Caron 2001)

46

Foundations Are Created in the Beginning

Relationships are like the planets—they move forward, but they keep returning to the same points. Relationships tend to orbit around their origins. If those origins were trust, love, and respect, then that will be the universe of that relationship. Without those positive values and feelings in the early part of the relationship, a sure foundation will be harder to establish.

WHEN IT COMES to love, Shawn doesn't take any chances. Instead of entrusting her romantic destiny to Cupid's arrows, the twenty-eight-year-old from Tampa believes in a more scientific approach. Shawn has turned to textbooks and tests and a marriage preparation course to guide her two-year relationship with her boyfriend.

"When we're on long car trips, I pull out my book and start discussing the chapters with him," she says. "At first he thought I was weird, but it has helped us examine the weaknesses in our relationship and to grow stronger."

Shawn says, "The best part is that we've been creating healthy habits from the start. Instead of letting a problem develop, and then having to try to undo some harm, we're trying to prevent problems and instill good communication. It's a lot easier to talk about something and head it off than it is to have to go back and undo something that has been going on."

Long-term studies of relationships find that the negative feelings expressed in the first year of a relationship can affect not only whether that relationship will continue on into the future but also whether or not it will be a happy relationship years later. (Huston, Caughlin, Houts, Smith, and George 2001)

47

Ambivalence Is a Negative

When we are not sure, we often put off making a decision. After all, we are worried we'll make the wrong one. This happens in all phases of life, including our relationships. The difference is that ambivalence about which shoes to buy doesn't affect the health of the shoes. Ambivalence about a relationship, in contrast, eats away at the relationship because it represents the absence of definite positive feelings—an absence both partners will be aware of. And that absence of a positive is a negative.

DOROTHY AND RICHARD were married in 1938. They were barely out of high school and were facing the continuing hard times of the Great Depression in southern Ohio.

"All our friends thought it wouldn't last," Dorothy said. "We were so young, it surprised us all. But, I guess, I was just young enough and dumb enough that I didn't have any doubts."

If the couple was foolhardy about anything, it was the economic realities of the time. "When we were married the first few years, things were tough, but we had each other," she said.

It was far from easy, Richard recalled. "When we got married, we didn't have anything. With our budget at the end of payday, we had fifty cents left over to spend. We went to the movies once or twice, but that was a luxury."

Richard continued, "It was a lot of hard work. But that brings you closer together. We just loved each other enough and stayed together. We never doubted each other, we never asked why we didn't have something. We had each other, and there was nothing greater than that."

One of the best predictors of future divorce among recently married couples is the expression of ambivalent feelings. Couples in which one or both partners mentioned any feelings of ambivalence were three times as likely to divorce within four years. (Huston, Caughlin, Houts, Smith, and George 2001)

48

Share Housework

It's unpleasant. It's not fun. Nobody particularly enjoys it. But the burdens of housework must be done. Relationships work best when both partners recognize these simple facts and embrace a sharing of the workload.

SUZANNE BIANCHI, a sociology professor, completed a major study of housework. She found that women shoulder the great majority of the burden. "We women have been brainwashed more than even we can imagine—probably too many years of seeing media women in ecstasy over their shiny waxed floors or breaking down over their dirty shirt collars. Men have no such conditioning. They recognize the essential fact of housework—that it stinks."

Professor Bianchi says that while neither men nor women want to do housework, women are more vulnerable to the situation. "If he begins to get bugged by the dirt and crap, he will say, 'This place sure is a sty' or 'How can anyone live like this?' and wait for your reaction. He knows that all women have a sore called guilt over a messy house. If he rubs this sore long and hard enough, it'll bleed and you'll do the work. He can outwait you."

Despite her deep knowledge of the subject, Professor Bianchi finds herself caught in the pattern. "If one person in a married couple wants more cleanliness and order, it still tends to be the woman. My calm comes from an orderly and clean household, so I do most of the work."

She does see one important trend that may change this relationship. It's not men doing more work; it's women doing less. "The path to equality, fortunately or unfortunately, goes through much less housework being done. In other words, you may not argue over who does the housework, but you'll be sitting on a pile of dust when you talk."

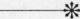

Couples who share housework duties report they are 19 percent more satisfied in their relationship than couples in which one partner does the vast majority of the work. (Allen and Webster 2001)

49

A Relationship Starts with Yourself

People need loving human relationships. We all benefit from close social contact. But many of us think relationships will complete us—fill in any holes in our lives. In reality, if you are not happy with who you are, a relationship will not change that, and in fact it will be difficult to maintain healthy relationships.

TESS, A MIDDLE-AGED accountant from Toledo, shares how her outlook has changed over time. "I used to see it as a chicken-and-egg problem. Which comes first, a healthy self-image or healthy relationships? It seems like you need a healthy self-image to have healthy relationships, and you need healthy relationships to have a healthy self-image."

She continues, "Then I realized that I had less control over my relationships—people up and move on you, or they enter new phases of their lives without you—so I had to start with myself.

"If you don't think you are a good person, worthy of your own affection, it is hard for other people to disagree with you. On the other hand, when I really looked for the value in myself, it was easier for me to see it in other people."

In long-term studies of middle-class Americans, those who were satisfied with themselves and their lives ten years ago are today five times more likely to report having a happy relationship with a love interest. (Paris 1999)

50

Let Go of the Burden of Pain

Y ou've been hurt and then apologized to. It is painful, but you decide it is within your heart to forgive. Yet the pain doesn't just go away. You carry with you the trauma of what happened, and you think of it even when there's no reason to.

You have to let go of the pain. Carrying it around makes it seem like the hurt is fresh every day. Only you can put it away. Ask yourself this: If you had to walk one hundred miles and had the option of carrying a massive cement block—a block of no value to you or anyone else—or carrying nothing at all, which would you choose? "Why would I possibly choose to carry this block?" you would ask. Exactly.

BEFORE HE left office, former president Bill Clinton said that he was focusing on "re-earning the trust and esteem of my family and the American people.

"While it is unusual for the president to be in a public situation like this, the fundamental truth is that the human condition—with its frailties and propensity to sin—is something I do share with others. And the most important thing about that is not that I can say, 'Oh, thank God I'm not the only sinner in the world.' Rather, it is that I can believe in the reality of forgiveness."

Clinton continued, "I think any time a person has to go through a searing personal experience and come to terms with truth, and genuinely

Gentle Reminder

from your dentist

Gentle Dentist
1121 West 2nd Street
Bloomington, IN 47403
812-339-1671

This is just to remind you that it's time for your next dental examination! Please call us at your convenience to schedule an appointment. Your last exam was February 17, 2010. We look forward to hearing from you soon.

02 1P
0003837519 JUN 30 2010
MAILED FROM ZIP CODE 47403
UNITED STATES POSTAGE
$ 000.28⁰
PITNEY BOWES

Yangfan Lu
2760 E Bressingham Way
Bloomington, IN 47401

atone, and genuinely make the effort to change, that's an immensely liberating experience. It makes you stronger.

"Seeking forgiveness gives me a chance to make my marriage whole, and my relationship with all my other friends whole, in a way that the keeping of secrets that are destructive cannot.

"Instead of wallowing in regret, I am working at repairing my life and my marriage. Wallowing in regret is a cop-out.

"Each day should be a new beginning. Personal and professional things happen daily to each of us, and many things can throw us off stride. The idea is to organize your life so you get back on course. I'm really looking forward to tomorrow and all the tomorrows because I feel freer than I have in a long time."

Studies find that those who have experienced a significant disappointment from their partner and have successfully granted their forgiveness to their partner are as likely to maintain a satisfying relationship as are those who had never experienced a similar disappointment in their relationship. (Alvaro 2001)

51

Develop a Healthy Calm

It is easier to maintain healthy communication if you are not prone to quick fits of anger. Maintaining your calm in stressful situations allows you not only to listen more closely to your partner, but also to think more clearly about the situation. While your inclination toward anger is in part a function of your personality, healthy habits such as exercising regularly, taking time out for yourself, and eating a balanced diet will lower your tendency toward lightning-quick anger.

"DO YOU KNOW that moment you've said something, and just as the words are leaving your mouth you wish you hadn't said it? I used to have that happen to me all the time," admits Tom.

"Unfortunately, thinking clearly is not required to talk. You can just open up and get started, only later figuring out what you should have said."

Tom was tired of the damage he was doing to his own relationship by saying things that exaggerated how he felt or were more hurtful than he realized. Tom started reading up on communication skills, not just in relationships, but also in high-pressure and stressful occupations. "I really began to see the dynamic at work. It was the 'you say something, I say something' contest. If you say something that knocks me back, I say something that knocks you back a little more. And then it grows from there. But what if you say something that knocks me back, and I don't say anything, I just think about it? Then I'm not as likely to come back at you and up the wattage of the argument. Instead, I might say, 'That was hurtful, but I want to address this problem for both of us.'"

Tom tried implementing his new communication strategy. "I didn't have any unrealistic expectations," he says. "I didn't think some switch was going to be turned on and everything was going to be better. But I think things are better because I'm doing less damage in disagreements, which means I can try to help with solutions instead of making the problem bigger."

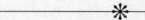

People who get angry quickly experience more arguments in their relationships, and their arguments continue 81 percent longer than people who are prone to remain calm. (Berry and Worthington 2001)

52

Think of Your Own Ideal

Think back to your first idea of what you wanted to be when you grew up. In grade school, chances are you wanted to be something you saw on television or have a job like one you came into regular contact with. These early career infatuations come and go and generally have little lasting effect on us. Now think back to the first image you had of the person you imagined you would marry. Again, the images come from things we were exposed to in the media or in our personal life. But, unlike our long-abandoned career dreams of becoming a ballet dancer or a football player, our images of ideal mates do not disappear as easily. For many, it is hard to shake the relationship expectations that surround us even if their origins were in the ill-informed imagination of a child version of ourselves. We must move past the images from our youth or from fiction and forge a relationship based on what truly matters to us today.

MICHELLE WAS SURE she had found the perfect man. "He had the right job, he had the right look, he had the right things. As far as I could tell, he was perfect." They married and started their lives together in Philadelphia.

Then reality set in. "He became more remote with each passing day. It was as if I were married to a photo on the wall instead of to a person."

As her marriage unraveled, Michelle blamed herself. "Then he was gone, and my self-esteem plummeted even further.

"I asked myself how this happened. Then I thought about what I really knew when this started. He looked the part. And if I'd hired him to be an actor portraying my husband, I suppose it would have worked out all right."

Five years later, Michelle is happily in a relationship, this time with someone she considers real. "I learned to pay attention to what matters. If you make a shallow decision based on what someone has to offer— money or looks—there's no reason to think they'll still have those things down the road. But if you find someone who has what really matters to you—a kind and generous spirit—they'll have that forever."

Research on marriages with high levels of conflict finds that more than half of these couples have disputes involving the failure of one or both partners to conform to popular images of husbands and wives. When partners discuss their personal expectations and feelings regarding what's most important, 38 percent of couples reported that the conflict in their marriage decreased significantly. (Philpot 2001)

53

Stay Flexible

D o you feel like you've had this argument before? People in relationships often realize that the same running themes, and the same patterns of conflict, appear again and again. The reason it happens is that people tend to adopt a means of conflict resolution within the first months of a relationship and maintain that pattern in subsequent years and even decades. The ability to maintain some flexibility in both your ideas and your habits will decrease your inclination to disagree and increase your ability to compromise.

A TEAM of professors from the United States and Great Britain recently concluded that "masculinity is in a real moment of transition."

What that means is that the behavior of young men and the preferences of young women are evolving. "I was really struck by the younger people's ideas," Professor Jane Pollins said. "They are responding to incredibly sensitive men who have real skills in conflict resolution—very different from the kind of tough, macho men who were once seen as the ideal," she said.

She sees younger generations as evolving differently from their fathers and grandfathers. According to Professor Pollins, "Men may have found a new emotional literacy that contradicts the traditional masculine stereotype but nevertheless is the man of the moment—sporting hero, style icon, and family man all rolled into one."

What interests Professor Pollins is that "this can create a supportive emotional relationship. Men who come into relationships with this kind of personal outlook tend to maintain it and bring forward healthier communication patterns for years to come."

When asked to describe the state of their relationship, those with a high level of rigidity in habits and thinking—that is, a resistance to new things, new ideas, and changes of any sort—named 38 percent more problems in their relationship than those who were more flexible in their thinking. (Kurdek 1999)

54

Think About Potential

In a relationship, we don't need everything to be perfect. We understand that there will always be challenges. What we do need is the constant ability to see the potential for improvement, the potential for resolution of difficulties. You do not have to solve every problem that comes up, and you should not strive for the complete absence of disagreements. But you must always keep part of your attention focused on hope, on the possibility that whatever difficulties arise today will be solved, forgotten, or at least less important in the future.

PATRICIA RECALLS returning to her home from work one evening to find her husband, Eric, sitting in the dark alone. "My life is over," he said. "I have no real purpose anymore."

A month earlier, Eric had taken an early retirement package and enthusiastically left his high-stress job. At the time, Patricia saw her own career as a consultant just peaking. "I understood that Eric missed his professional environment, the prestige of being an authority in his field, and even the business travel he used to complain about so much," she says. "He used to get phone calls from all over the country asking for his advice with business problems. Now I'm asking him what he's making for dinner."

She continues, "Did I throw my arms around him and say, 'Oh, poor darling'? Certainly not—I kicked and screamed and threw things.

The truth is, I took his unhappiness as an insult. After all, he was married to me."

Researchers at Cornell found that many who retire from jobs—even jobs they didn't like—express feelings of aimlessness and disappointment in the subsequent months. They recommend that people plan for transitions in their life—expect pain even in positive transitions—and allow for a period of discomfort. Those in relationships should discuss role changes, new divisions of labor, and new purposes if they wish to stay focused on the possibility of positive change and the hope that the relationship will continue to meet their needs.

Eric found his stride a few months later. "I saw that I have fewer stresses and demands than ever. Any stress I have it's because I choose to have it," he says. "There's a great deal of happiness if you look for it. I can see that now," he says. "That was the life we led and enjoyed then; this is the one we enjoy now. The common element is that even though my life has changed, my love for Patricia and my true purpose remain the same."

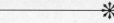

A strong belief in relationship efficacy—that the relationship can continue to move forward and meet both partners' goals—is an aspect of nearly nine in ten relationships that continue successfully into long-term commitments. (Thomas 1999)

55

Even in a Relationship, You Are Still an Individual

Strong, healthy relationships are built on notions of equality. With that comes the realization that the individual matters. When two people are in a relationship, chances are each is pursuing individual dreams. The strongest relationships support both partners' dreams, even if they differ, not one partner's at the expense of the other's.

LANA AND DEREK moved in together seven years ago. They had been seeing each other for a year, but before they moved in together they sat down and carefully discussed how money and household duties would be handled. Thus far their system has worked well: they split everything fifty-fifty.

Lana says, "We try very hard to strike a balance between being together and letting both of us individually be the person we want to be. I work for a large company, and I'm a bit of a workaholic; he's an artist. So at times we're both on our own running around doing the things that make us tick. But we both understand that our work can only bring us so far and that sharing with each other makes it all more worthwhile.

"We have a strong commitment to each other, which I think will last because we also have a strong commitment to ourselves. Because I think that's what makes a relationship commitment sustainable."

Eighty-eight percent of people surveyed reported that maintaining their sense of individual autonomy, their own independence and equality, was an important factor in their relationship decisions. (Thornton and Young-DeMarco 2001)

56

Rest Up—This Is Going to Take Some Effort

All the behaviors that foster a strong relationship, that produce happiness in the moment and in the long run, require not only effort but an ability to see things from your partner's perspective. All this effort is far less likely to take place when you are exhausted. Realize that rest is a required ingredient for you and your partner to find your time together satisfying.

KEITH GULPS COFFEE all night long. "Sweatshop is a good description," the veteran long-haul truck driver, husband, and father of four says, describing his job. "But I've got to do it. I'll probably kill myself putting my kids through college. But there's no way I'm ever going to let them drive a truck.

"We drive hard, putting in long hours day and night, often for not much more than minimum wage. And we have to drive tired, pushing mile after mile on a few hours of sleep, sometimes just to break even. We get paid by the mile, not by the hour. We get paid for delivery, really, not for what's necessary in between."

Truck drivers often spend weeks away from home and family, living out of duffel bags and sleeping in the back of their rig. "I know guys who are running so hard that they haven't been home in two months.

Some are on their third and fourth marriages. One of my friends says the only thing he's got left is his cat and a truck.

"My wife wants me home here for the weekend, but the company's got me headed in the opposite direction. When I do get back, I'll be so tired I wouldn't notice it if the couch were on fire. I'll sleep for a couple days then head out for my next run. And my wife will say I wasn't ever really here."

Driving 130,000 miles a year, sometimes up to a hundred hours per week, Keith has come to one conclusion: "Something's got to change."

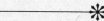

People feeling excessively tired found that they were more likely to experience conflict in their relationship and 25 percent more likely to feel emotionally out of control. (Roberts and Levenson 2001)

57

Like the Way You Look

If you are not comfortable with your image of your body, you will not be comfortable with anyone else's image of your body. And if that happens, it will erode your self-confidence and make it much more difficult to find or maintain a relationship. Although it's not terribly logical, people equate body imagery with all kinds of unrelated powers. And those with the positive images assume positive outcomes for themselves. You need to separate out the media images of the perfect body, which almost no one has, and focus instead on healthy habits and positive thoughts.

ANYONE WHO'S EVER had a bad-hair day knows how it undermines self-confidence. Now a psychology professor's research confirms this.

"Bad-hair days affect self-esteem, increasing self-doubt, intensifying social insecurities, and making people more self-critical in general," says Professor Marianne LaFrance.

And bad-hair days affect men, too, her study found: troubled hair makes women feel more disgraced, embarrassed, ashamed, or self-conscious, while men feel more nervous, less confident, and more inclined to be unsociable.

The study, which had an ethnically diverse group of young people fill out psychological tests, found that just the thought of a bad-hair day caused both men and women to feel they were not as smart as others.

Professor LaFrance warns, "We talk about self-esteem coming from the inside, but the reality is much more complicated than that. In our culture, how we look affects our sense of self and our ability to take action in a very powerful way."

In surveys of American adults, people rated those with attractive bodies as having a 59 percent greater chance of having a good marriage and a 48 percent greater chance of having a successful career than those with less attractive bodies. (Bush, Williams, Lean, and Anderson 2001)

58

Don't Romanticize the Past

We tend to have positive notions of the past. Times were simpler, life was easier, families were stronger. Admittedly, definitions of family life have changed tremendously in the past fifty years and divorce rates are higher now. But the traditions of the past included marriages based on almost no existing connection between the partners and, in the case of a loveless union, the expectation of lifelong suffering because there were no available alternatives. While we face challenges in finding and keeping relationships today, we should also see the opportunities and the freedom available to us that did not exist in the past.

MICKEY ROONEY is a living piece of show business history, having performed since childhood and now past an age when most people would be retired.

The variety show he still performs around the country is a retrospective of his career and his life. He is joined onstage by his wife, Jan Chamberlin Rooney. And through film clips of his previous work shown to the audience during the performance, he's joined by many of his seven previous wives.

While the temptation to be melancholy about his personal life is great, Rooney takes delight in celebrating his life and loves. He admits to the audience that his life was empty before he married his first wife, Ava

Gardner. He then adds, "Married life with Ava was great. Boy, could she cook. Ever had fried water?"

As he pokes fun at the checkered course of his relationships ("I've been married so many times I've got rice marks on my face" or "Alimony is like pumping gas into someone else's car; I've pumped a lot of gas"), he also dedicates the show to Jan Chamberlin Rooney. At the end of the show Jan and Mickey sing "Let's Call the Whole Thing Off" before he sheepishly asks her if she'll put up with him for one more day.

Studies comparing relationships today to relationships fifty or more years ago find that levels of commitment are largely unchanged, but the biggest difference is that freedom of choice to enter, maintain, or leave relationships was less prevalent then. (Medora, Larson, Hortacsu, and Parul 2002)

59

Share the Praise and Share in the Blame

Whether we mean to or not, we tend to give ourselves credit for things that go well, and we tend to blame others when things go awry. A disagreement was the other person's fault. A wonderful night out was the product of our own efforts. Understand that you are likely to see things this way and your partner is as well. If we can learn instead to graciously accept some of the blame and generously share the credit, we will be contributing to a happier relationship.

"I'LL TELL YOU my relationship philosophy," says George. "It comes down to two phrases: 'I'm sorry' and 'Thank you.' If you overuse those two phrases, things will go smoothly. If you use them when you think you should, there will be many bumps along the road. If you use them less than that, you won't make it very far." People keep asking George for answers because he's been married over sixty years.

"I love my wife and always have. We enjoy being together. It's a recognition of being proud of somebody. You're willing to help them to make them happy," he says. "We've just never fallen out of love, and we do things together. We just would never think of divorce. We're probably a one-in-a-million couple. I just would never think of living with anyone else but my wife. She's a sweetie," George says.

But George, like many others married during that time, faced tough challenges. He says their commitment to each other made it easier to surmount those challenges. "Because it was so easy being married, we could better handle the hard times when others were turning against each other because it was so easy to do," George said.

Because he had no money to spare, George's first Valentine's Day gift to his wife was a stick of gum. "And you know what? She said it was the best gum she'd ever had."

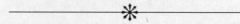

In interviews about their relationships, people were three times more likely to emphasize their partner's role in problems and twice as likely to emphasize their own contribution to the strengths of their relationship. (Johnson, Karney, Rogge, and Bradbury 2001)

60

You Can't Find Without Looking

The vast majority of relationships start after meeting in school, at a workplace, in a common neighborhood, or through family or mutual acquaintances. While you may find the partner of your dreams in these places, typical sources are also tremendously limiting. If you are looking for someone, think carefully about where you look and how you can expand your interactions with new people.

KAREN SAYS that on a whim she sent in a personal ad to her local Rhode Island newspaper.

"My girlfriends and I would read the ads and kind of laugh," Karen says. "I never even considered that that would be something that I would do." However, Karen was tired of the people her friends tried to set her up with, so she decided to give it a try.

"You can leave it to happenstance and serendipity to meet someone, or you can be more active about it," Karen says. "It's just so convenient. It's a lot more immediate."

And, more important, "After all the responses I received, it gave me a chance to pick from among the possibilities. A number of them I clicked off immediately because either their tone of voice or what they said was a turn-off to me," she says.

One of the responses Karen received led to a date at a bookstore. Karen and Mark talked for hours. Shortly thereafter, they were meeting for dinner a couple of times a week. "It's probably fate," Karen says. "Relatively quickly after we started seeing each other, we felt like we had known each other for a good long time." Less than a year later, Karen and Mark were married.

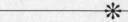

Among those who have used a personals service, 73 percent thought the effort was worthwhile. Users said the best feature of the service was that it exposed them to people they would never have met otherwise. (Kalmijn and Flap 2001)

61

Meaningful Commitment Is
Mutual Commitment

Your efforts alone, no matter how great, cannot make a relationship healthy or satisfying. A relationship not only requires effort from two people but requires mutual effort from two people. Increasing your commitment to your relationship will not help unless you do so with your partner. On a rowing team, everybody has to try hard, but no one can try harder than anyone else or the boat will go in circles. The same is true in a relationship.

DRS. JOHNNY AND PEGGY Emberson of Georgia gave up their practices. His was obstetrics and gynecology and hers dental. Instead of continuing lucrative careers in the United States, they headed off together for Nepal, where they would donate their skills as medical missionaries.

"You always get more than you give," says Johnny of donating one's time and effort. Peggy says she and her husband just want to use their gifts to the best of their abilities.

The Embersons work out of a hospital in Kathmandu, the capital city, and also help train workers in rural areas. Peggy said only a small percentage of the population has medical care and that the country has a high infant mortality rate.

How did they make such a momentous decision to give up not only practicing medicine in the United States but also living here? "We are equal partners in everything we do. It is how we started together, and it is how we continue together. Johnny put me through dental school, then I put him through medical school. We were partners on this decision 100 percent. You would have to be, of course. One person can't very well decide to send a couple to Nepal, but because we're on equal footing and both dedicated to each other, we can both make a sacrifice for each other, and for a greater good, and feel right about it."

In studies of the health of relationships over time, the most stable and successful relationships did not feature the highest level of total commitment from partners but close to the same level of commitment from each partner. (Drigotas, Rusbult, and Verette 1999)

62

Friendships Predict Relationships

While they are obviously not as intense, close friendships require the same foundation of communication skills and selflessness necessary for a successful relationship. The requirements of being supportive and willing to adapt over time are necessary for both. Take the confidence you have in your friendships, and understand that if you can maintain a friendship you can maintain a relationship.

TEACHERS BETH AND MATT both bring a wide assortment of friendships into their relationship with each other. They met at the elementary school in suburban Maryland where they both work, and they got married there as well. Beth invited her current and previous first-grade classes to the ceremony, and both she and Matt, a physical education teacher and coach, included their colleagues in the event.

"The thing I love the most about her is really the way she treats other people," Matt says. "She just really is one of the genuinely nicest people I have ever met, whether she is dealing with students, peers, friends, or anyone. You can see in the way she treats people that she takes joy in all kinds of relationships."

Beth sees Matt's treatment of other people as one of his strongest points as well. "Matt is loyal," says Beth. "He is loyal as a friend and colleague, and in teaching you have to be loyal to your kids. And, of course, loyalty is important in a relationship."

People with strong social skills, including an ability to maintain long-term friendships, were 32 percent more likely to be satisfied with their relationship. (Flora and Segrin 1999)

63

Prepare for Milestones

I n long-term relationships, we often think of today as an extension of yesterday and tomorrow as an extension of today. We may not particularly notice how time is passing or pause to reflect on our circumstances. Milestone events, however—births, deaths, career change, children leaving home—inspire reflection. These events encourage us to look at ourselves and our relationships and often lead us to question the path we have taken. This experience is jolting because it is unexpected. Reduce the significance of these occasions by taking time to reflect on your life whether or not a milestone event is at hand. And give yourself time to adjust to the aftermath of an event. Don't make important decisions in the wake of a major disruption.

NEW YORKERS Carol and Bill were, in their own words, coasting through marriage together. When their two sons moved out of the family home within weeks of each other, both Carol and Bill fell into a deep contemplation of their journey together.

"We both realized we were getting worn out," said Bill. "We kept running into the same arguments and roadblocks. It was getting tiresome."

Carol added, "We had kind of fallen into mediocrity, like, 'Ho-hum, this is it for married people.' The passion, the electricity, the vibrancy of being in love were in the past."

They decided to attack the problem of their relationship being on cruise control. "When Bill and I came to the disillusionment, we said, 'We have a decision to make. We can continue down that road, or we can decide to love each other.' It's like taking the first step to get by an impasse. It's the memory of how good your love was once before that helps you want to make it better."

To heal the distance they felt between them, they decided to take twenty minutes every day to do nothing but share their feelings about everything from the world to each other. Sometimes they write each other notes. "When you are just getting started, there's always a nice or sometimes inspiring note being written. Twenty years later the only note you'll get says 'buy milk at the market.' We decided to change that.

"I vowed my life to Bill forever, that he should be my number one priority," said Carol. "When you put everything into perspective, twenty minutes a day is not that radical to improve your life."

Bill is also excited with the direction their relationship has taken. "I do wish we had woken up to this long ago—that we hadn't waited to be shaken out of our patterns."

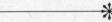

In the aftermath of a major life event, people are eight times more likely to question the health of their relationship than they are in general. (Schwartz 2000)

64

Don't Bring Your Job Home with You

We spend more waking hours on the job than doing anything else. We are taught from a young age to value hard work and that it will be rewarded. We hear far less about the efforts required in our relationships and the rewards that will come to us based on those efforts. Working at your job as hard as you possibly can is not working as well as you possibly can. When the workday is over, the work must recede out of your thoughts and time.

JAMES KELLER DESIGNS home offices—spaces in existing rooms or entire rooms dedicated to working from home. He thinks the home office concept is a metaphor for the home office worker.

"The space I design has to serve two functions. It has to be a home part of the day and an office part of the day. When you think about it, that's just what the person is, too—a family member part of the day and a worker part of the day. This is a limitation in a sense, since the design has to incorporate both functions. But it is also a strength because, done right, it serves the greater need."

Keller strives to make the space something that exceeds people's needs instead of something that just minimally functions. "I don't want to make a design that people can suffer through; I want to make something people can enjoy—someplace you want to be."

Keller's concept of a home office is not a space that beckons you to the office at all hours of the day. "You have to turn off the office lights and shut the door and then see your house as a home come five o'clock. You might say, 'I work in that room from nine to five. Come five o'clock, I'll clean up, and it becomes a family room again.'"

One of the easiest and most important things Keller advises is to use storage units. "Pack it up and put it away at the end of the day. That keeps your work safe from mishaps and misplacement." It also helps put the person in the right frame of mind. "Just as important, packing your work away moves you into the next phase of your day."

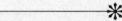

Workaholics, people who never seem to stop working or thinking about work, are three times more likely to say that their personal life is unsatisfying. (Porter 2001)

65

We Assume Similar Preferences

It's difficult, sometimes very difficult, to figure out what other people are thinking and feeling. As a shortcut for doing just that, we look to our own thoughts and feelings and assume that the other person's are pretty close to our own. The danger in this habit is clear. Our feelings are not representative of everyone else's, or anyone else's, for that matter. When, lacking better information, we project our own feelings onto someone else, we wind up offering our preferred response to our own projected feelings. While we assume similarity because it is easier to do so, if we were being realistic we would more carefully consider others' preferences.

IF OPPOSITES ATTRACT, thermally incompatible couples are a case in point. You know the ones: she's cold in layers upon layers of clothing, while he's sporting shorts and a T-shirt in January. It's a common problem. The important thing is how they deal with a situation over which, for meta-bolical reasons, two people may have little control.

No matter what he does, Tim can't seem to keep cool. His wife, Mary, is always cold. "I turn the thermostat as high as I can bear it, and she sits there wrapped up with a blanket, sweatpants, and a sweatshirt," Tim said.

Mary watches television downstairs by the fireplace, while Tim might watch the same program upstairs, where it is generally cooler. That compromise usually gets them to bedtime, when Tim ratchets the thermostat downward and Mary sneaks in behind him to bump it up. "It's kind of funny to watch the two of us," Mary said. "It's like a covert operation to change the thermostat. 'Are you touching the thermostat? No,' we say, lying."

Mary Lou Murray, clinical psychologist, says that many couples have trouble seeing things from the other's perspective. "When we're warm, we just don't understand how at the exact time and place, someone else could just as easily be cold. We have a lot of expectations that begin and end with our own perspective—when to eat, when to sleep, what's a good temperature. These are matters of individual preference, but they often get applied to couples. Each person has to be respected, though. Each has to understand that what is strange to you about someone else is likely strange to someone else about you," she said.

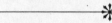

Across both relationships and friendships, more than eight in ten people assumed a similarity of reaction between themselves and others in rating things they liked and disliked. (Watson, Hubbard, and Wiese 2000)

66

Don't Let Secrets Eat You Up

While honesty might be thought of as the best policy, some truths might be too devastating to admit in a relationship. On the other hand, the burden of a secret weighs on us and may force us to live with consequences of our dishonesty that are larger than if we had told the truth. In situations in which you fear that the effects of the truth in your relationship might be devastating, seek a trusted confidant with whom you can discuss the truth and relieve your burden.

THEY WERE SEPARATED. If she told the right story he'd never really need to know. She says she didn't even know what she was doing when she was caught.

Doreen had become mixed up with the wrong people, and when she delivered a package for one of them, it led to an arrest and a six-month jail sentence. With her marriage in tatters already, she thought surely this would be the final straw. But she decided that telling the truth might do her some good. It was a hard thing for her to say, telling her husband, Eric, that she was heading to jail. But it was liberating. "The more I put it out there," she says, "the less power it has over me."

Doreen dreamed of the moment she would be free and could return to her native Alaska. She imagined landing at the airport and being swept up in hugs upon arrival. After so much time "swallowing silent tears in dark places," as Doreen described it, she cried when she saw

Eric waiting for her. "He's the only person in my life who's willing to get his hands dirty and help me."

An aspiring poet, Doreen won a poetry competition just weeks after her release.

"She's inspiring," Eric said of his wife. "She's just really talented. I always knew she had the talent to do it." She persevered in the belief that she could overcome the cost of telling the truth, the cost of the truth, because, she says, "In a world so bleak, I needed idealism to stay on my feet."

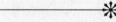

Among people who have held important secrets from their partner, 27 percent report having had feelings of physical sickness from the discomfort of the deception. (Kelly and Carter 2001)

67

To Find a Better Way,
Look Where You've Been

Humans tend to be creatures of habit. We repeat the same behaviors over and over again, often without much thought or reflection. It's why we tend to buy the same brand of soap over and over again, even though there's little difference between the brands. It's also why we tend to repeat much of our behavior with regard to relationships. Sigmund Freud argued a century ago that, good or bad, the model for our human interactions was cast in the experiences of youth and was likely to be repeated throughout our lives. Unless you make an effort to think about what you are doing and why, you are likely to repeat yourself, often to the detriment of your relationships.

WHEN FORMER SPEAKER of the House Newt Gingrich told his second wife he had been seeing another woman and wanted a divorce, he didn't mention that the affair he'd started had been going on for six years. "I found out with the rest of the country watching a news conference held by his lawyers," said Marianne Gingrich.

Marianne was shocked. "This is about a marriage. This is not about politics and another press conference. This is about my life," she said. Marianne has found it hard to speak of the end of her eighteen-year marriage and her husband's affair. "I don't have any way to express it."

She later found out that the affair began "at a time of great vulnerability for me." According to the time line her husband's lawyers produced, Newt's affair began while Marianne was shuttling between the Gingriches' homes in Georgia and Washington, D.C., and her mother's home in Ohio, where her mother was suffering from a terminal illness.

"I can tell you that Marianne thought that they had a very sound marriage, right up until this unexpected demand for divorce," her attorney said. He noted that Newt Gingrich served his first wife with divorce papers while she was in the hospital recovering from cancer surgery. "Mr. Gingrich has a very disposable view of people, of loved ones. When they no longer serve his purposes, he trades them in. From what I understand, this has been his practice all his adult life."

People who said they had strong feelings of personal security in youthful relationships are 31 percent more likely to be socially supportive in their adult relationships than are people who did not feel personally secure as a child. (Lawrence 2001)

68

Money Matters Less over Time

If you were purchasing a house, you would pay attention to the features that matter most to you. But when we are thinking about potential mates, we pay the most attention to things that matter the least to us in the long run. That is, when we conjure up images of the ideal mate, that person is often pretty wealthy. However, when we actually live our lives, the significance of wealth drops to almost nothing in our evaluation of our relationship.

AS AN EXERCISE to get his students to think about what really matters to them, Professor Todd O'Brien asks them about their parents' dreams. "Did you ever ask, 'Dad, if you could do anything with your life and it didn't have to involve income, what would that be?'"

What he finds are countless stories of dreams deferred and forgotten. "What would your parents have done differently if they had not let money make decisions for them?" the professor asks.

He tells them of his own background. "My dad spent all his life working in the accounts department for a corporation. It was sort of a drone job. He talked about getting an apple orchard in Washington. But he never did. I never forgot about that apple orchard."

Then Professor O'Brien asks the students how much their parents talk about their lives in terms of financial outcomes. "Do they talk about the dollars they made—the money that passed through their hands?"

After the students focus on the imbalance of the role of money in their parents' dreams and lives, Professor O'Brien tells them, "You may think that your life will be built on money and that your relationships will be built around money. But the things that will sustain you, that will give meaning to your life and your love, have nothing to do with money."

Given only data about income, it is impossible to predict the likelihood of a relationship's success because wealth is unrelated to relationship length and satisfaction. (Kenrick, Sundie, Nicastle, and Stone 2001)

69

Recognize the Value of Shared Values

Your core values were formed a long time ago and will likely be yours for the rest of your life. The same is true for the other person in a relationship. Given that neither of you is likely to change your core beliefs, it helps if those beliefs are compatible. Strong relationships depend on trust and communication. Trust and communication are fostered by shared values. When you have similar beliefs, it feels safer and more rewarding to share your thoughts and feelings.

AS HER HUSBAND put it, "Some people enter a room and the entire area seems to light up. Jane is definitely one of those people. She is vibrantly alive."

When Jane Douglass White was thirty, she had life in the palm of her hand. She was happily married, the mother of two healthy children, and the associate producer of the network TV show *Name That Tune*. The songs she had written were sung by such well-known vocalists as Julius LaRosa and Eartha Kitt. Jane owned and managed an off-Broadway theater, sometimes staging shows using her original scripts and music. "The sky was the limit," she thought at the time.

Then the words of the physician cut like a knife through her consciousness.

"You have cancer and must have surgery immediately." It felt like a death sentence because, at that time, White knew no one who had recovered from cancer.

Although he was wracked with fears, her husband offered her comfort and strength throughout the long ordeal of treatment. To White, her recovery was nothing short of a miracle, a miracle she could never have endured without the steadying hand of her husband.

"He saw what was most important—that we both lived in love instead of hate; in forgiveness instead of resentment. And that no illness could change the fundamental bond of our lives together."

The degree to which couples have similar values does not change over the course of their relationship. Those with similar values, however, are 22 percent more likely to rate their communication habits positively. (Acitelli, Kenny, and Weiner 2001)

70

Understand What You're Looking For

People have basic ideas about the world and their place in it. These ideas are fundamental to their life and to everything they do. To better understand what you need from a relationship, think about who you are. Your interests, beliefs, career choice are all indicators of your fundamental personality. Remember, your choices about things other than relationships reveal a lot about what you need from a relationship.

THE WORKDAYS get tougher leading up to Valentine's Day for Debbie. She manages the marriage license office in a southern Maryland county. And she gets a variation on the same frantic questions again and again leading up to the big day.

"'Are you going to be open? How long do we have to wait? Can we come in and get married?' We've been getting swamped with calls from folks," she said. "We say, 'Yes, we'll be open and ready for business,' and you can almost hear the relief."

Her work reaffirms her feelings about her own relationship, though. "Helping people in the process of joining together really lets you see the joy inside them. It is a daily reminder of what is important to them and to me."

"I couldn't live without that kind of faith and hopeful spirit. And my husband is the same way. He looks at the bright side of things—and jokes that there's a reason he married someone in the marriage office and not the divorce office."

People's occupational direction was among the best predictors of their views on relationship roles, with those in nurturing professions such as education and medicine being 47 percent more likely to take a nurturing view of their relationship role. (Klute, Crouter, Sayer, and McHale 2002)

71

Never Let Faults Stand for the Whole

People in longtime relationships have a distinct habit. When asked about their partners, they don't bring up a long list of complaints. It's not that their partners are perfect, but their tendency isn't to dwell on faults. In fact, people in long-term relationships not only spend much more time thinking about the good traits of their partner but also tend to see redeeming features even in the faults. These people see the complex reality that is another person and recognize that within everyone are both admirable and regrettable qualities but that within most of us the admirable qualities predominate.

RODDY CLEARY has performed dozens of civil union ceremonies since a historic bill went into effect in Vermont allowing gay and lesbian couples to have their relationships recognized by the state government.

Cleary has officiated at ceremonies on a farm, in a restaurant, in a state park, and in the Unitarian church in downtown Burlington where she is a minister. Her husband, William, also performs civil union ceremonies.

Roddy and William describe themselves as "wildly, madly, insanely in love." Married for thirty-three years, they see their role as helping other couples come together and demonstrate their love. "Uniting couples in love strengthens our society. Gender is incidental; differences can be a source of strength. That's how we look at it in our marriage and in our work," Cleary says.

When officiating at a civil union ceremony, Cleary tells participants, "To be able to share in another's joy is what heaven is about." She says she became an outspoken advocate for the civil unions in part because of her experiences for fifteen years as a campus minister at the University of Vermont. She worked with "outstanding gay and lesbian students who were gifted, beautiful people who had, by virtue of being gay, gone through a difficult identification process. The relationships that come out of all that suffering," she says, "are so tested and refined that they ultimately strengthen the fabric of our society."

Cleary sees both her own marriage and her participation in other unions as the ultimate expression "of seeing the good in people. Glimpsing the good that we are all capable of.

"I received a letter from a man who didn't want his daughter to marry another woman, but he wrote me afterward and said, 'Your sense of spirituality, your obvious pleasure in addressing our daughter's spirituality, enhanced our joy.' And I think, maybe for the first time, he saw some good in his daughter's marriage."

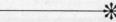

People in long-term relationships spent five times as much time talking in response to a question about their partner's positive qualities as they did talking about negative qualities, and tended to qualify comments about negative qualities by explaining away their importance. (Murray and Holmes 1999)

72

You'll Need Some Relationship Friends

Two people in a relationship bring with them many friendships from their past. While undeniably important, these friendships do not always fit well into the context of the relationship. Sometimes the lack of common interests and common backgrounds stilts communication, and at times jealousies erupt between friends and partners over your attention. In addition to your personal friends, then, you should try to form some relationship friends—other couples with some common interests who can interact as a couple with you and your partner. Relationship friends help ground us in the importance of our relationship and give us a fun and healthy outlet for activities built around other people but that include our partner.

BEFORE CHRIS got married last August, he regularly spent a lot of time with his single friends. "They thought I was crazy when I got engaged," said Chris. "Before we got married, or got serious, I would have rather hung out with them because I didn't know how things would go with our relationship. But after we got serious, I hung out with her. The relationships with them ventured off because she's my best friend."

Sherry Welch, a psychotherapist who has studied friendship-relationship issues, says the dynamics within the relationships of a dating couple and their single friends usually change quite a bit once the couple gets serious. "Any meaningful commitment between the couple tends to exclude others, at least for a time," she said. "Some of it depends on the maturity of the couple as well as the single friend. The friend can feel left out and abandoned, depending on what the couple does to include him or her."

Chris says that is what happened in relation to some of his friends. "I'd say my best friends are more jealous than mad, but mad 'cause I don't come by as often as I did," he says. "My friends get mad when I choose my wife over them, and I don't think they understand when you marry somebody they have to be your best friend. That's how I was raised.

"We've got a couple of married friends now," Chris says. "That's something we talked about and decided we need to have some people in our lives who don't react to our relationship but want to be our friends, as we are, together. It's sad when people's roles in our lives are reduced, but we can't let anyone undermine our lives."

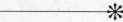

Among those in a relationship, satisfaction was about 3 percent higher for each couple they regularly socialized with. (Cox 2001)

73

Don't Wait to Start Moving
in the Right Direction

We tend to miss a lot of opportunities to think about things, to make changes, to make things better. We often continue down the path we are on regardless of whether we find it rewarding or even acceptable. It's as if our lives are just a series of school days, one after the other, in which we show up where we are told and do what we think we are supposed to. We know someday there will be a graduation, when we will do something different, but until then we continue without question. Don't wait for the moment that shakes you out of your routine to examine what you are doing. Work on making your personal life as fulfilling as you want right now.

HE WAS A PROMINENT and wealthy Texas surgeon. He appeared in television ads for his medical clinic. While holding his daughter in his arms, he looked into the camera and said, "We treat you like family."

When she first met the surgeon, Colleen was awed and delighted by him. He dazzled her with vacations in Europe, ski trips to Colorado, and an African safari. "He told me that he wanted me to quit my job, that he loved me, and that he would support me. And we would just go have fun, travel, and everything would be great." When he proposed, she accepted.

Colleen says her new husband quickly became more and more controlling, insisting she drop plans for college and demanding she begin carrying a cell phone so he could reach her instantaneously. Within a year, they had sought marriage counseling to try to work out mounting disagreements. Fights had become frequent. Romance, according to Colleen, had been replaced by an increasingly oppressive routine.

After a separation, the two eventually reconciled, and there was new hope for the marriage with the birth of a daughter. Instead, the relationship began spiraling into violence. After one particularly bad incident, Colleen called the police. Immediately she regretted it. She told her husband's lawyer about the call, and he told her to make up a story. "I had to sit there and lie through my teeth," recalls Colleen.

The pattern continued for more than a year. "I realize now, of course, that I was blaming myself for things I couldn't control. And indulging this fantasy that he would change." When the doctor, without telling Colleen, decided to change the locks on the house while Colleen was out of town, it symbolically proved a point Colleen was struggling with. "He thinks he owns the house, me, everything in his life. And that will never change."

Colleen divorced the doctor and successfully sued him for inflicting physical abuse. "I'm stronger now than I ever was with him," concludes Colleen. "I hope he gets help. But he hasn't taken responsibility yet for anything he has done."

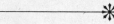

Researchers found that more than nine in ten people in mentally or physically abusive relationships blamed themselves for contributing to the situation, and that self-blame was a significant factor in delaying their efforts to change or end the relationship. (Hilfer 1999)

74

Music Can Bring Us Together

Think about a situation in which a couple is on the brink of being irritated with each other. Maybe they had a hard day, or maybe one said something that could be taken the wrong way. They sit there uncomfortable, the silence between them magnifying the tension. And then one of them puts on their favorite album. The music permeates their thoughts. The tension dissipates, and both partners are put in mind of shared joys and good times. Music can enliven and transport the mind, and music shared between two people can be an important and healthy form of communication.

"WHEN YOU'RE OLD, people think either you've lost your nut or you've got some special knowledge. Here's what I have: You have to give and take," Herbert, ninety-three, says. "And obey the golden rule."

"And forgive each other," adds Elsie, his wife, who is ninety.

The two met as teenagers at a local dance. The attraction was immediate, but their courtship lasted more than a year. "We went to a lot of dances," Elsie said.

The couple spent nearly all their married life struggling on a small Missouri farm. It was a hard life but a happy one, the two agreed. She remembers the treeless prairie, sandstorms, and blizzards so severe a rope was needed to move safely from house to barn. The family burned cow chips for fuel. For many years their home had no electricity. "We could only spend a nickel once a year for ice cream," she says.

"I tell a lot of people how we had it and they don't believe it," her husband agrees.

"I always had a piano, though," Elsie recalled. "And he played the violin. And you know what? I'd start playing and he'd start playing, and the next thing you know we're teenagers at a dance again. It never fails."

In counseling sessions, exposing a couple to music of their own choice increased feelings of cooperation and caring in seven out of ten people. (Housker 2001)

75

Define What You Need

We start a relationship with high expectations. Yet, for many of us, the traits that grab our attention, that make us think a relationship would be worth pursuing, are not the same things that will meet our needs and make us happy over time. Think about what you truly need from a relationship, and let that guide your relationship goals and decisions

"THEY SAID it was the opportunity of a lifetime," John remembers. "It was a promotion, a chance to run my own division, but it was also a transfer a thousand miles away."

John turned down the promotion to stay in his current position. "It was flattering, but it doesn't make sense right now." Why? His wife, Liz, was immersed in the struggles of a first-year medical residency.

Liz works twelve-hour days and spends every fourth night on call at the hospital. The Charlotte, North Carolina, couple has to pull out their calendars each month to coordinate a few hours of free time together. "It's kind of pathetic, but we have to get our schedules out, and I'll ask him what's a good day to take off," says Liz.

When she finally could take a week off, the couple went all the way to Africa to escape the pressures of work. They went on a sightseeing safari vacation in the Serengeti, known for its lions, giraffes, and other exotic animals. "It was neat to see John in a place where it was hard to get in touch with his office," Liz recalls.

But Liz was inspired by John's decision to defer his own career path. "It's ironic, because what I first found exciting about John was his ambition and drive. And now what I find most exciting is that he's put that aside. It is really a testament to what's most important to him. He understands the meaning of our life together, and when my training is completed, I will move wherever he'd like to go."

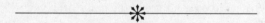

Researchers found that the traits that first attracted people to their partner were no longer relevant to 34 percent of them when asked six months or more after they began dating. (Felmlee 2001)

76

Show You Care, Even When It's Hard To

In a perfect world there would be little or no conflict in a relationship, and it would be easy to show you cared every day because you would be happy and eager to do just that. In the real world, you will likely experience many disagreements and points of conflict in your relationship, and it is hard to show you care when you are in the midst of a conflict. That said, it is also vital to do so. In fact, there is no more important time to demonstrate that you care, that you value your partner, than when difficulties arise. Even as you disagree, never fail to recognize and to show what matters most to you.

DURING GROUP RELATIONSHIP sessions, counselor Peter Dilliard explains that each person in a relationship must invest time, energy, and interest in the other one. "If you're not willing to invest in the people in your life, love will not grow. Investing in someone means caring about that person's feelings as part of your day-to-day life and understanding their needs, and doing so right in the middle of a disagreement about right and wrong, money, time, anything at all," Dilliard says.

"The relationship investment involves sacrifice," Dilliard tells participants, "even though the word is not usually associated with relationships. Sacrifice is doing something you don't want to do because it will make the other person happy.

"No matter how hard it gets, you don't withdraw, emotionally disengage, and stop investing in the relationship," Dilliard says. "You can't be a rock and be loved. You must open up and be vulnerable. Love grows as you make the other person feel special and invest in the other person."

Dilliard draws some looks of disbelief when he declares, "If managed properly, conflict can bring a couple closer together." He says that if you focus on the solution, not on the disagreement or on who is at fault, "a conflict becomes a way of demonstrating commitment, love, and understanding. It becomes a way of demonstrating the strength of the relationship, not the weakness."

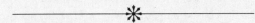

When couples experience conflict, they are 45 percent less likely to feel pessimistic about their relationship if they can recognize feelings of caring from their partner during the disagreement. (Ebesu Hubbard 2001)

77

Make Your Decisions for Positive Reasons

Most people tend to have avoiding negative outcomes as their top priority when making decisions instead of making decisions by seeking the positive outcomes of their choices. In relationships, this means that we tend to ask ourselves what's to be lost if I make this decision instead of what's to be gained. This pattern can lead to continuing unsatisfying situations because of a fear that things might get worse. Make your decisions based on getting what you want, not on avoiding what you don't want.

NOT TOO LONG ago, Ali was giddy. She'd met a great guy, and she was so confident in the relationship's future that she moved in with him after just a few weeks of dating.

The couple was engaged a few months later and got married at city hall. "We knew that we were going to be together," Ali said.

"It was good at first," she added. "We worked well living together. But me being in the same space with somebody—it just became like two dogs in a cage together." Ali said she was too free spirited to fit into her husband's orderly existence. "It was something we would have discovered anyway, but living together so soon didn't help," she said. "We didn't have that initial buildup to the relationship. We threw ourselves in, and we did that by living together."

Still, the cage, as she called it, was comfortable for a while.

Even though they were both unhappy, neither sought a change. "We had just bought a house, so that made it hard to walk away. Then I didn't look forward to saying to everyone I knew and to my family that I'd made a big mistake. Especially when I knew some of them had been shaking their heads from the start."

They continued living together for six months after she had decided the relationship was broken. Then she gave up. Reflecting back on the experience, Ali said, "I've learned not to be in such a rush—and that you can't keep a relationship alive merely for convenience' sake."

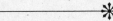

In a study of those whose relationships had faced feelings of betrayal or serious disappointment, people who continued a relationship for negative reasons (fear of losing their relationship) were overwhelmingly unsatisfied with their relationship (61 percent) or had discontinued their relationship (24 percent) six months later. (Roloff, Soule, and Carey 2001)

78

A Relationship Is Built
on a Foundation of Support

If you believe your partner supports you—supports who you are, supports what you are, supports what you want, and supports what you need—your relationship is built on solid ground. Any disagreement that might arise is ultimately less important, and any difficulties your relationship might encounter are conquerable, if you start from a position of mutual support. Give support and demand support in your relationship, and everything else will be easier and better.

THEY WERE a typical couple, part of a nuclear family that included young children. Since both were career minded and ambitious, they had made an agreement early in their marriage: Denise would put Jerry through school, and then he would help her while she went to school.

Everything was fine—until Denise began her graduate school studies. Jerry shirked his share of the housework and child care duties. He began to complain about how much money her studies cost the family.

When Denise confronted him about his behavior, Jerry said that he hadn't realized that her studies would be so hard on him, that she'd be gone so much, and that he'd feel so neglected.

Then Denise graduated and began earning more money at her job, only to have more problems arise at home.

"Jerry felt like the balance of power in the marriage had been changed, and he was somehow devalued now because I was making more money than he was. He began to see himself as a failure," says Denise.

Psychologist Warren Reed has seen this problem with increasing frequency. "Rarely do careers progress in tandem," Reed notes. "More often than not, one partner's career is taking off while the other's is in a temporary holding pattern. Working late and not having time for family often creates tension and resentment. If a couple doesn't plan how they'll work through the stresses of nonparallel career paths, they will likely experience relationship problems.

"Many of the men I spoke with admitted that although they'd been committed to an equal relationship at the beginning of their marriages, they found it difficult to maintain their open-minded stance, particularly when they felt their wives weren't giving them the kind of attention they wanted," he says. "Many act out when they feel they've lost a sense of control that defines their masculinity."

If a woman tries to overcompensate for her husband's dissatisfaction, he says, "that is where we get into this 'superwoman complex'—doing everything right in the office and then doing everything at home. It's self-defeating, because now he resents her for being more perfect."

Reed advises couples that "both partners need to see the value of the support they have received from each other. They need to see that their connection to each other outweighs these feelings of unflattering comparison."

Researchers studying couples placed in stressful situations found that when both partners felt support from the other, they actually experienced less discomfort, with supportive couples showing 38 percent less effect of the stress on their blood pressure and heart rate. (Harris 2001)

79

The Pieces of Your Life
Must Fit Together

Your two favorite foods might taste delightful separately but terrible in combination. Chances are, you plan your meals carefully to get the combinations right. Your career and your relationship, likewise, are two forces that combine to make your life. Seek not two ideals that would never fit together but two compatible situations that will make your life work.

JANE IS A COACH. A life coach. Based in Portland, Oregon, she helps clients throughout the country reach their goals in everything from efficient use of time to career planning and even life satisfaction.

She holds weekly meetings, sometimes in person, sometimes over the phone or by email, with her clients, to discuss how they are seeking fulfillment and balance in such matters as career, family, health, hobbies. Jane boasts that the right coach "may not help you find anything you weren't going to find eventually, but a coach can take the learning curve down from forty years to two years." Jane says that comes from two factors: "helping people find their focus" and "highlighting the future and what it has to offer."

Despite enjoying the work immensely, at one point Jane realized something was missing. "I spent my time guiding people to their own fulfillment and then woke up one day and realized I wasn't heading toward mine." She evaluated where she was and, with the help of her own coach, decided to seek a better balance between her work and her personal life.

"I still think about my clients and do the best work I can for them, but at some point each day I have to completely stop that. I help people pursue their dreams, but to keep doing that, I have to pursue mine, too."

More than seven in ten professionals report that their job has stood in the way of a satisfying personal life at some point in their career. (Gilbert and Walker 2001)

80

Master Your Fears

Social interactions, whether talking to friends, meeting someone at a party, or being with a partner, require you to reveal something of yourself. For many people, this process is nerve-racking because we fear that what we say and do won't be good enough and will be cause for rejection. People overcome these fears in one of two ways: either they come to believe that everything they say and do will be adored, or they let themselves not care about winning everyone else's approval every moment of the day. Abandon the fear of negative reaction and the need to edit yourself moment by moment because those who react positively to the real you are the people whose company you should seek.

"HOLIDAYS MAY BRING out the best in some people, but they bring out pain for many others. People tend to hold unrealistic expectations of what the holidays will bring—lingering kisses under the mistletoe, the perfect gift from their soul mate, and declarations of love rivaling Romeo and Juliet," says Professor Susan Brown.

"Commitment seekers often use the holidays to mark the progress of their relationship and mistakenly assume that if they're together for the holidays, they're together forever," Professor Brown says. "They tend to analyze every detail and judge the relationship by what does or doesn't happen, what is or isn't said, fearing that if their expectations are not met the relationship is doomed."

But Professor Brown warns, "In this situation, people sabotage their relationships, or their chances to start a relationship, because it's the only way they can breathe. They will pick a flaw, change plans, become difficult or argumentative. They seize opportunities to create distance.

"So many relationships stumble at this time because people want so much, they fear they won't get it; then they can't have anything. Thanksgiving, Christmas, and New Year's are three hits, one after the other."

Professor Brown says, "Feelings of fear and doubt should be acknowledged but not acted upon. Give yourself permission to feel uncomfortable and not be perfect and not do the holidays in a perfect way. Do not try to be the perfect partner. Just give yourself permission to be a human being. You will see your fears are unfounded, and you will give yourself a chance to have what you want."

Fears in social interactions such as meeting new people, or speaking in front of a group, afflict more than nine out of ten people. Researchers find that these worries can be reduced for most people through positive visualization—imagining the interaction before it happens and seeing yourself in a positive role. (Honeycutt 1999)

81

We Are All Much More Alike Than Different

When we think of people, we often focus on their differences. We see different groups, different religions, different ethnicities. We imagine these different groups do things quite differently from us. But the struggles and hopes that characterize our notions of relationships are the same as countless others'. Do not allow surface differences to overwhelm your acknowledgment of inner similarities.

Bev and Sil face challenges that might overwhelm anyone. As a lesbian couple, they are not allowed to legally marry. Without being married, Bev, an American citizen, and Sil, who is from England, cannot obtain the family waiver that the U.S. government offers to provide citizenship to the foreign spouses of U.S. citizens.

"I do not know when I will see my beloved again because our love and commitment is not recognized or respected by the laws of the United States," Bev says.

"As we all are painfully aware, it doesn't have to be like that. Usually governments allow and even encourage binational couples by making immigration relatively simple for them. It is not too dramatic to say that we are actually being forced apart by our governments." Bev and Sil make extended visits to each other, but they cannot legally stay together in the United States beyond six months.

"I often read that the majority of the American people oppose same-sex marriage. I cannot imagine that many of them have stopped to consider the extremely cruel impact of this discrimination on our lives," Bev says. "When I hear this appalling statistic rattled off as though it were just one more factoid with no particular meaning, I think of the fact that only thirty years ago, laws against interracial marriages were finally struck down by the United States Supreme Court as unconstitutional. I try to imagine how it must have been for an interracial couple faced with the prospect that their love was outlawed, their human dignity trampled on, and their lives made much more difficult by such an oppressive system.

"And yet, the truth of the matter is, the irony of all this is, we aren't any different from any other couple. We love, honor, and respect each other like any other couple should. We have arguments, get on each other's nerves sometimes, like any other couple, and we want nothing more than the same chance any other couple has to face up to the challenges of life and a relationship."

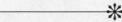

In how they viewed relationships, in their fears and feelings about relationships, and in their conceptions of ideal relationships, all ethnic groups in the United States showed similar responses. (LeSure-Lester 2001)

82

Limit Your Interest in the Past

We all are curious about our partner's past. We want to know about all their previous relationships, and especially the serious ones. But too much attention to this subject is dangerous. It breeds worry, comparisons, and ultimately conflict. You are not in competition with past partners—and they won't be a part of your relationship unless your feelings of jealousy or worry let them in. There is nothing you can do or say that will change the history of your partner, but by not harping on that history, you can make the future of your relationship stronger.

SOMETIMES, THE RIGHT time is a half-century in coming.

High school sweethearts Veta and Jess met in the early 1940s. War raged in Europe as Veta and Jess were finding love on the home front. He was a year ahead of her in school in rural Arkansas. They were good friends before the attraction deepened. She was just fifteen, and her parents wouldn't let her go on car dates until she was sixteen. "I thought I would never have that birthday," she recalls.

But before long, Jess's birthday would alter their lives. Jess was drafted when he turned eighteen. He soon found himself flying B-17 bombers over Greenland.

"I told her I didn't want her to be tied down," Jess says. He wanted her to be free to see other people while he was gone. Three years later, Jess received a medical discharge and returned home. Veta, however, had married someone else. "I was heartbroken," Jess says.

Jess would later marry—and remain happily wed until his wife passed away forty-eight years later. Veta was happily married for forty-seven years, until her husband died.

Jess and Veta kept up with each other over the years through mutual friends. "I just always wanted to know how she was doing," Jess says.

They also kept old high school pictures and love letters from each other. They say their spouses knew of the past relationship, but they gave their spouses no reason to be jealous. "We respected each other and each other's spouse and the decisions they had made. And that's the end of it. No what-ifs or looking back wishing for something else," Jess says.

"We both loved and married very good people," Veta says.

Within a year of each other, Jess's wife and Veta's husband both died. Jess became extremely depressed. "I couldn't think of or find or see any hope," he says.

Several months later, Jess and Veta renewed an old friendship. Then an old romance. "I thought I was going to faint," Veta said, recalling their first kiss in five decades.

When they later married each other fifty years after their first date, there were no regrets for the circuitous path they had traveled. "We had wonderful lives separately, and we're going to have a wonderful life together now."

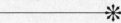

More than two in five people report that jealousy over a previous relationship is a source of conflict in their current relationship. (Knox and Zusman 2001)

83

Get Your Reality from Reality

Many of our images of relationships come from the media. The power of these media images is in the fact that we see them all the time but give them little thought. We watch a television show or a movie for entertainment and spend little time wondering about the way a person was depicted or questioning the stereotypes about men and women that we saw. Question this silly information before it becomes your basis for understanding.

"WHOEVER SAID LOVE conquers all hasn't watched television recently," says sociologist Richard Grier. "At one time, TV was filled with people in lasting, loving relationships: Ricky and Lucy Ricardo, Heathcliff and Clair Huxtable. But on today's shows commitment is fleeting and happy marriages are rare."

A study of people in their twenties found that many expected to be single for a very long time as they sought someone worthy to marry. "It provides a very unrealistic view of what marriage really is," Grier said of that finding. "The standard becomes so high, it becomes easy to bail out."

Indeed, Grier said that bailing out, or not even taking the plunge, is the primary love message of many television shows.

He points to the typical representation of a successful man on television today. "Frasier Crane, first on *Cheers* and then on *Frasier*, was jilted repeatedly when he was a Boston barfly, then had an unhappy marriage.

After a divorce Frasier moved to Seattle, where he finds fault and failure with every woman he meets.

"When you look around now, it's really hard to find a realistic role model," Grier says. "Most characters treat relationships as throw-away items. The few long-term couples, such as on *Everybody Loves Raymond*, seem not to particularly like each other." And it is not very funny to Grier that the couple with the longest-running marriage on TV is Homer and Marge Simpson.

"My overall viewpoint on almost all relationship issues is that it's darn complicated. Most of television is about sound bites, and that model for communicating is at odds with what it means to be human," he says.

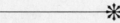

Heavy television watchers were three times more likely to subscribe to stereotypes about men and women and were quicker to make assumptions about people than were those who watched less television. (Ward 2002)

84

You Are Never Too Old to Find Love

People give up all the time on relationships because they think they've run out of time. The truth is that the need for human companionship does not go away over time. Neither does the capacity to find joy in a relationship fade over time. Never give up, because you are never too old.

ROMANCE ELUDED Shirley during her youth. Her marriage was a great struggle in the face of a terrible tragedy.

Her first husband broke his neck soon after their wedding, rendering her a full-time nurse for three decades until he died. He was a nice man, but theirs was not a satisfying relationship for her. At sixty, Shirley found herself a widow, primed for a new companion, hopeful that this time she might discover all of love's reward.

Undaunted by the many years since she'd last gone on a date, Shirley drafted a list of requirements: He had to be under seventy-one, energetic, and spiritual. No smoking, no facial hair. He could drink socially but not to excess.

"I think the second time around you should be more fussy," she said.

Jeff was a recent widower. Friends dragged him to a seniors' outing at the local roller-skating rink.

Shirley noticed him immediately. "Oh, I have to find out who this man is," she thought. "We breezed by each other and said hello and introduced ourselves."

At the end of the event she extended herself a bit further. She told him she was glad he came and hoped he'd come back. That was it—one smiling signal of interest that kept him coming back to a steady stream of senior mixers and socials.

Now they've celebrated their fifth anniversary together. They swim, walk, dance, take trips, and, of course, roller-skate. "My darling husband prepares breakfast daily and does so many thoughtful things like bringing me flowers often," Shirley says. "Loving and being loved is the greatest gift in this life. And it can happen to you anytime."

Studies show that people expect their love life to reach its peak in their twenties or thirties, but relationship satisfaction is higher among people in their sixties than among people in their twenties. (Koehne 2000)

85

We Look Inward to See How People Feel About Us

What information would you want to know to figure out if a person felt well liked and well loved? Would you ask about their relationship? Would you ask about their friends? Would you ask about their family life? While all these indicators of social support are important and contribute to life, the biggest indicator of feeling liked and loved, surprisingly, does not depend on relationships with other people. That is, the health of a relationship or the number of close friends—the outward indicators of being liked and loved—are not as important in predicting a feeling of being liked and loved as is self-esteem. People who like themselves feel liked and loved regardless of the state of their relationship and regardless of how many close friends they have. People who do not like themselves do not feel liked and loved even if they have a healthy relationship and many supportive friends.

PSYCHOLOGIST MARTIN PUGH teaches self-acceptance in counseling sessions and workshops. He says it's a trait we can't live without.

Pugh tells the story of a patient living a passive life. "Shuffling into my office, he had all the charisma and mastery of a timid dog just in from the rain. Everything he said oozed accommodation and inferiority. 'Is it all right if I sit here?' 'I hope I'm not wasting your time with this.' 'I'm not very good at this sort of thing.' "

As Pugh delved into his patient's situation, he heard about a series of unhappy relationships, unmet dreams, goals that had come and gone, and a daily life of worry, conflict, and endless second-guessing.

"What do I need?" the patient asked. "Medication? A support group?"

"Power," Pugh replied. "You need your power. The vital and sustaining power available to the individual, the power that emanates from the human spirit."

Pugh says, "Wherever you probe psychologically with someone with personal power, you hit something solid. They're always home and always grounded. Although strength of spirit is available to each of us, many never tap in and bring it to the forefront of their lives. Some simply don't believe they possess this vitality. Its presence doesn't fit with their self-image of being quiet, passive, or ineffectual.

"In my experience, the overriding reason people fail to bring forth their personal power is the absence of self-love, a compassionate self-acceptance, psychological warts and all. Like many of life's major challenges, the answer is simple: love thyself. But the execution can be taxing. Primarily, it is accomplished through an act of will, a heart-felt decision to speak the truth, live one's beliefs, risk pursuing one's dreams, and embrace the good in oneself and others."

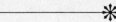

People with low self-esteem devalued the degree to which other people saw them positively regardless of the strength of their relationships or the number of friends they had. (Murray, Holmes, and Griffin 2000)

86

Be Willing to Evolve

Few things are more frustrating than realizing you are reliving a problem you've already had to deal with. When the same conflict keeps coming up in a relationship, both partners will feel frustrated and trapped by the disagreement. A relationship therefore requires that both parties be willing to evolve. That does not mean giving up the traits that define you, but it does mean adapting your life to reflect your commitment to your relationship. And it does mean avoiding rigidity in your thinking. If you can put yourself in your partner's place and learn from that experience, you will evolve in ways that make possible a better relationship.

RICHARD ANDERSEN is a man with a mission. A former mapmaker, pastor, restaurant manager, and retreat center leader, and now a financial planner, he is helping people align their faith, values, and finances.

He says that too many people are resistant to change, even when their present condition is untenable. "My whole life was kind of a struggle to break free from other people's expectations and get clear about mine," he laments.

While he has enjoyed all of his jobs, Andersen discovered that he "really wanted to be active, not passive, in people's lives. I wanted to help them uncover their passion and live more integrated lives."

He's convinced that he has found exactly that in his work with the LifeMap program, which brings together a team of professionals to help people see clearly their life priorities and integrate their faith, values, and finances. His team helps clients identify core values and then examine how a change—an attitude change, job change—might bring them greater joy.

"For a lot of us it's the realization that we've been pursuing our parents' dreams and it's time to go after our own," he said. "It's easier to stay the same than it is to change. But staying the same comes with some big risks we sometimes don't recognize."

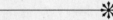

People who are rigid in their personality and thinking—that is, highly resistant to change—were 42 percent more likely to report a high level of conflict in their relationship. (Eldridge 2001)

87

Connect, See You're Capable, and Know You Count

E ach of us has a few core needs that must be met if we are going to fit into human society. We must see that we are connected to others—that we are not alone and that our decency is unshakable. We must see that we are capable of accomplishing important goals and making a contribution to the lives of those around us. We must see that we count—that we matter in the grand scheme of things. Each of these beliefs is central to being able to have a relationship and being able to maintain a relationship.

MOST PEOPLE WOULD be scared to take a job that required them to gain twenty pounds. Most actresses, surely, would worry their career would be jeopardized by the idea of gaining twenty pounds in order to play a woman whose thighs wobble when she cavorts in a Playboy bunny costume. But Renee Zellweger, who did just that to play the heroine of *Bridget Jones's Diary,* claims it was "a thrill for me. It was so much fun. I felt strange only in that I felt alien to myself sometimes. I've never been that heavy.

"Weight is a very personal journey," she continues. "It's unique to each woman's experience and her own way of defining her self-image and self-worth. It's a wonderful theme in this film. Through the mistakes you make and the ones you face and, in Bridget's case, with a sense of humor you have self-discovery and self-acceptance.

"Growing up, I never heard, 'Oh, you're so pretty.' It was never about looks. It was about, 'Anything you want to do you can do.' I'm lucky that I don't have those messages floating around my head from an early age of trying to match some expectations that had been projected onto me from childhood."

When seeking a relationship, she says, "it's important to know your boundaries. What you have to keep in yourself, things you must know without question. Just for purposes of survival, and to be real instead of superficial."

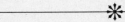

People who felt connected, capable, and that they counted were twice as likely to feel positive about their relationship and that they were contributing to their relationship, and they were less than half as likely to worry about their body image. (Conway 2000)

88

Reliability Counts a Lot

With all the complicated advice available about relationships, sometimes the basics can be overlooked. Relationships depend on communication; we all know that. And meaningful communication demands reliability. Your words need to mean something. Say what you mean, and do what you say you are going to do. Always. If you do, you will have taken a huge step toward positive communication and a positive relationship.

WHEN PRINCE EDWARD'S engagement to Sophie Rhys-Jones was announced in Great Britain, it was a dream come true for the couple and the royalty itself.

For a royal household eager for a little good news, the announcement of the prince's engagement to his girlfriend of five years produced great joy. Buckingham Palace displayed a rare level of emotion, describing the queen as "delighted" and "thrilled" about the first royal wedding since 1992. Indeed, far too many royal weddings have led to the unfolding of royal indiscretions and royal divorces, followed by royal revelations. Each of the queen's other children, Anne, Andrew, and Charles, has endured a much-publicized marriage breakup. This unhappy cycle has become all too familiar to the royal family and the world.

Then came Sophie.

The announcement captured the front page of every newspaper in the country plus the first seven to eight pages inside, which were filled with more Sophie photos and stories putting out the details of the new family member. In what the press called "an exquisite twist," this thirty-three-year-old public relations professional was "far from flaky—already a break from tradition—and she was widely proclaimed as relatively normal," a word not often used on the royal beat.

Unlike the typical princess, Sophie does not come from an aristocratic background; she was raised in a farmhouse in Kent. Her father is a former car salesman who later worked for a tire company.

Newspapers looked on the addition of a regular person to the royal family as a wonderful step forward. "They're happy, madly in love, and it might just last!" one paper wrote. Another put it this way: "Even in this cynical age, few events are more capable of brightening the gloom of a British winter than the prospect of a royal wedding. After years of turmoil and personal tragedy, perhaps the palace can at last look forward to a new beginning." Her friends said they were confident this relationship would prosper. "She's real and true, and will give her all to this," one friend said.

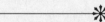

People who consider their partner conscientious, a person who consistently does what they say they are going to do, were 26 percent more likely to rate their relationship healthy and reported 41 percent less conflict in their relationship. Dependability was rated among the most desired qualities in a partner. (Watson, Hubbard, and Wiese 2000)

89

You Are Complete by Yourself

A relationship is not a requirement. Your health and welfare do not require a relationship. A relationship may be a crucial part of your life and your future, but you by yourself have everything necessary to survive and thrive. Believe in yourself—regardless of your situation right at this moment—and you will be complete.

"LONELINESS IS a universal experience known to every human being on Earth—single parents, teenagers, and even the happily married. Even the rich and famous suffer from loneliness," says psychologist Henry Abrams.

"Polls show more than a third of all Americans feel lonely in an average week. Many more of us probably have feelings of loneliness but are reluctant to admit it, feeling ashamed and stigmatized by our loneliness and seeing it as a sign that we are unlovable or defective instead of recognizing occasional loneliness as an essential part of the human condition."

But Abrams says that despite what many assume, surrounding yourself with people is not a cure. "Loneliness stems from a void within ourselves, a sense of feeling incomplete and unfulfilled even when we have many loving people in our lives.

"To feel complete, we need to nurture a strong connection with our inner selves. Then we can more fully connect with others and find their company rewarding."

Abrams warns that feelings of loneliness often lead to behaviors, such as excessive sleeping, television watching, or computer use, that serve only to distract for a moment but make us feel worse in the end. Abrams's advice? "Don't take feelings of loneliness as a reason to further isolate yourself."

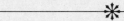

People who are not in a relationship are not lonely by definition. In a study of people currently seeking a relationship, the reported frequency of feelings of loneliness varied from always to never. (Fahrenkamp 2001)

90

Intensity Fades

Ahigh-intensity relationship produces both heights of happiness and depths of despair. Over time, relationships generally produce both fewer complaints and fewer feelings of rapture. Recognize the easy trap of fading intensity, and fight it with regular reminders to your partner of the depth of your feelings.

"WE ARE a quick-fix society. When we are tired of something, we get rid of it. Sustaining a relationship requires overcoming this tendency that we practice in all other aspects of our life," says psychologist Drew Raines.

Professor Raines demonstrated the effects of the newness principle with a simple experiment. He gathered more than one hundred volunteers and placed them two at a time in a room together. One person was to say something the other was known to disagree with. The disagreements were over matters of opinion ranging from their rating of the president to what's the best restaurant in town. He then tested the reaction of the other person. Did this person openly disagree? Did she or he do so politely? Was there friendliness even in the face of the disagreement?

The crux of the experiment was that in one version of the test, the two people in the room had never met before, and in the other version the two people in the room were in a relationship with each other. Professor Raines found that "with total strangers, people could be decorous and polite. They restrained criticism; they did not jump down throats of strangers; they respected each other's opinions or at least pretended to." But with their partner, people "would disparage what the other person would say; they were most discouraging, and they didn't stint in their criticism.

"Collectively, this means we really are clueless about how to treat each other. Day after day, most of the mean, caustic, angry, evil things you will ever say to someone" are to a loved one, he said.

Professor Raines explains this pattern: "As the loss of illusion sets in, we become bored. Our inclination to sacrifice for the other is reduced, and we wind up engaging in negative behavior we would not even consider with a new person in our lives. We have unmatched opportunities to cause grief in a relationship, and we have to work even harder over time to see that we don't take up those opportunities. We need to work to rediscover our relationship, to rediscover the joy. Then we can capture the feeling of newness, of beginning again."

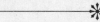

Studies of married couples find that as time passes, couples have fewer disagreements and fewer episodes of difficulty. At the same time, long-term married couples express about 1 percent less excitement and less marital enjoyment per year of marriage. (Kulik 2001)

91

Beware Second Opinions

In almost anything we do, we are taught to value informed opinions. The best decisions, we think, are made after hearing from multiple sources. We often get a second opinion when an important decision has to be made. Relationship decisions are, of course, important, and many of us seek the input of those we trust. The problem with this strategy is twofold. First, no one else can assess what we truly need and value in our personal life. Second, people tend to be far less optimistic about the relationships of others than they are about their own relationship. In other words, the people you talk to are more likely to see the negative than the positive in your relationship. When it comes to relationship decisions, you'll have to decide for yourself.

GLEN TAYLOR is the billionaire owner of the Minnesota Timberwolves basketball team and the Taylor Corporation. Among other things, the Taylor Corporation is by far the largest wedding invitation printer in the United States, with 50 percent of the total market.

Taylor kept a hectic business schedule running his company, but he also had a passion for politics. "I was listening to various people who told me what was important, told me to run for governor. Said I could put my family aside for the moment.

"My wife said she would support my decision to run. But while I was in politics, my marriage needed me full-time. My marriage was falling apart. By the time I looked up, it was too late to save it."

While Taylor is disappointed that others' advice hurt his family life, he ultimately blames himself for listening to it. "I was romanced by this idea people were putting in me." He calls the neglect of his marriage "the worst misstep" of his life.

A decade later, Taylor talks of keeping his priority on people and relationships rather than on money. And he's learned to ignore the advice of others when it comes to what is most important to him. "I think we all have to listen to our inner thing," Taylor says. "I pray that I don't make my decisions based on ego and don't listen to others when I should be listening to myself."

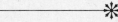

Four out of five people say they have had to ignore others' advice to maintain their relationship. In fact, when asked to rate their own relationship, people were 23 percent more likely than their family members to think their relationship would continue happily into the future and 17 percent more likely than were their friends. People's optimism about their own relationship turned out to be more accurate, as their predictions were more likely to be true than were those of family or friends. (Boyer-Pennington, Pennington, and Spink 2001)

92

Have Faith but Don't Forget Reality

Americans are wildly optimistic people. When asked about almost any topic, most Americans think they have an above-average chance of having something good happen to them—everything from success at the job to winning the lottery to being unusually happy to buying a house that will increase greatly in value. Optimism is a big factor in starting relationships and in increasing our level of commitment. Optimism is culturally ingrained, and it's not going anywhere. That said, we cannot let optimism set us up for disappointment. Faith that things will work out should not lead us to think every day will be perfect. Believe in others and in the future, but believe, too, in the work it will take to make that future what you want it to be.

"THERE IS ONE thing I wish all brides would have on their bridal registry: a marriage skills course," says Diane Solle, founder of the Coalition for Marriage, Family, and Couples Education in Washington, D.C. Solle, who counsels couples, worries that people seek help when they've encountered trouble in their relationship instead of avoiding the trouble by seeking help at the outset of their relationship.

What is the single biggest problem Solle sees? "Unrealistic expectations about how wonderful and easy it's going to be. Couples are operating under this really crazy notion about finding Mr. and Mrs. Right, and they think that's somebody they're not going to argue with."

One of the most important skills for all couples, she said, is to understand there will be bumps and rough spots along the road. "We need to shift our perspective from looking at marriage as 'I've arrived now; everything is fine' to 'This is an opportunity to build our relationship and to grow.'" Solle favors an up-front dose of reality from day one. "The marriage vow should say: 'I agree to disagree with you for the rest of my life. You're the person I'm going to discuss and argue and work things out with forever.'

"What I tell people mostly is to look at time as an ally. You're talking about lifelong relationships. There's no urgency to get everything right and running smoothly in the first few months. Everyone needs time to readjust to the new role. The couples who make it to the finish line are going to learn to understand that differences are normal, even good," says Solle.

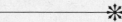

Studies of people seeking a relationship and studies of newly married couples found that more than nine in ten expected their relationship to be unusually happy in the future. (Fowers, Lyons, Montel, and Shaked 2001)

93

Pay Attention

I mportant problems often have complex, difficult solutions. The most important problem in a relationship—the failure to communicate—has a simple solution: pay attention. The first step in understanding someone else's viewpoint, in responding to their needs, is paying attention to them. The single biggest stumbling block to being attuned to a partner's emotional status is not paying any attention to it.

"AFTER TWENTY-ONE years of marriage, Craig left me for a younger woman, an administrative assistant in his office," says Kelly, a bank executive and mother of two grown children. "He said we were in a rut and he had to do something different."

For weeks, Kelly couldn't eat; she cried herself to sleep each night. Then Craig showed up on her doorstep begging forgiveness.

More than anything, Kelly was in shock over the course of events. "Craig was always so calm and so patient. We never fought."

Kelly had suspected something might be wrong when Craig started coming home from work later and later. "I'm not sure he was happy at work," she remembers thinking. But she did not pursue the subject or ask Craig about his feelings.

At that point Craig felt his entire foundation was coming loose. "My life had gone sour in every way," Craig explains. "Until they brought in this younger guy over me, I'd had a lot of responsibility and liked my job. Next thing I know, I hate it." At home he didn't feel appreciated, either. "Kelly was busy with her work, her friends, she could barely squeeze me in. Then when I wasn't there, she would nag me. The more she nagged me about not being there, the more I forgot to comply. There was never any room for fun."

Craig's feelings of powerlessness at the office and then at home finally erupted. Craig turned to a younger woman who made him feel appreciated. Mistakenly, he thought that the only way to make his life happier in the future was to make a complete break with his past.

Kelly and Craig both now realize that had they been more aware of each other's feelings and the stress points in marriage, they might have been better able to understand their feelings and work through their problems.

For now, they are trying to save their relationship. "Of course, I love him," Kelly said, "but I can't stop thinking about the other woman. And I can't just erase all the pain."

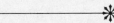

Researchers have found that there are no major differences in the ability of men and women, or of long-term and short-term couples, to judge the emotional state of their partners. The difference lies in the effort expended to do so—which is 26 percent higher in moments of distress than in more typical times. (Ruef 2001)

94

Nice People Don't Finish Last

It's a popular notion to think that nice people are overlooked, while other people have all the fun. The implication is that you shouldn't be nice if you want to find a relationship. In truth, the quality of being nice is among the most highly valued in potential partners.

KIM IS A social worker in Chicago. "I met this guy through a friend's husband. They were co-workers, and I was set up on a blind date. I was a little hesitant at first because I had never been on a blind date before and I wasn't quite sure what to expect."

Kim tells how the blind date unfolded. "We spoke on the telephone a few times and had good conversation. He was very much into music. I told him I like all kinds of music, but I was getting more and more into jazz. He invited me on a jazz cruise, and I accepted. He seemed kind of nice, so I bought a bottle of cheap champagne and two plastic cups for the date and slipped them into my purse.

"When I got into his car, he had a bag and told me I could look inside if I wanted to. It was Moët and real champagne glasses. I laughed to myself, but I didn't tell him why. It was a nice surprise. I never did pull out my $7.99 bottle."

She continues, "When we got to the pier, we opened the champagne and had a toast to new friendships and new beginnings. The boat ride was romantic. It ended around 10 PM, but we stayed on the pier until

1 AM talking and laughing. It was so nice. He was not trying to kiss me or anything like that. It was just a nice wholesome date with a nice guy."

Looking back after three years of marriage, Kim remembers her trepidation about the blind date and says, "Don't let anybody tell you there aren't any nice guys out there."

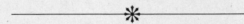

Among those seeking a relationship, the degree to which a potential partner was nice and kind was a significant factor for more than 75 percent of respondents. (Herold and Milhausen 1999)

95

Relationships Are like Modern Art

While successful relationships have many things in common, much of the time our assessment of the state of a relationship is purely personal and unrelated to specific events or factors. In other words, what you see in a relationship, like what you see in a piece of modern art, depends on how you look at it and what you are looking for. Don't be limited by others' ideas and viewpoints in evaluating what you have and what you need.

"YOU CAN'T HAVE what someone else has. You just can't," says Elaine, a nurse. Unhappily married in her twenties and happily married in her forties, Elaine has learned something about perspective.

"I wish that I had known somebody I could have talked to before I got married. I thought of marriage almost like you would buying a house. You pick one out you like, something maybe like a friend has. Then you buy it, and it's yours."

Of course, she says, "it doesn't work that way. Marriage is more like you buy the materials, and now you have to figure out how to use them, how to build something with them.

"What I learned through experience is that I had to figure out what I wanted for me and not for anybody else. You have to take the burden off yourself of trying to recreate anything. Instead, you will be better off creating your own unique relationship for you and your partner."

Studies of happily married couples found that in more than half of all couples, idiosyncratic factors such as personality compatibility and habits, aspects that varied from marriage to marriage, were important to understanding marital satisfaction. (Bachand and Caron 2001)

96

It's Not Easy, Even if It Looks It

Wᵉ all know someone who seems to lead the perfect life, with the perfect love. We've all seen countless movies with perfect love stories. The truth of the matter is that relationships are work for everyone. There are no perfect love stories, although there are many stories of dedication, devotion, and a willingness to work through the hard times. Everyone struggles through difficulties finding or maintaining their relationship.

WHEN JUAN AND MARIA and their three sons moved to Ohio, their new neighbors thought a perfect family had moved in. But Juan and Maria knew their ten-year marriage was on shaky ground.

"From every appearance, we had it all together," Maria said. "We went to church. We got along with each other in public. We were involved with our kids' lives. But the truth was, Joe and I were struggling to maintain the image. We lacked any real connection with each other. We spent nearly all our time blaming each other for just about everything.

"It was as if divorce was calling ahead to say we should anticipate a visit," Maria said. "And in my heart I knew it wasn't just Juan's fault. I was equally to blame. But I had trouble keeping that idea in the middle of an argument."

With pressures at work and at home, tempers reached a boiling point over a forgotten credit card payment. "We were screaming at each other about this payment and everything else. Tears were rolling down both our faces. And I said that I couldn't do this anymore. This bill isn't more important than life," Maria remembers.

Both Juan and Maria sought counseling and have worked hard to adopt a new approach to each other and to their lives. "Keeping our marriage on a positive track is not a piece of cake," Juan admits. "But it's amazing how much easier it is when you remove the land mines from self-centered lives. Maria and I are learning to keep better standards with each other."

Researchers found that more than nine in ten people could name someone they considered to be an ideal couple and that most felt disappointed they could not match the couple's relationship success. (Taylor 2001)

97

Most People Are Looking for Experienced Rookies

The subject is inevitable: "Tell me about your previous relationships." What most of us want to hear is neither an endless saga nor a short story. We are most comfortable with a partner who has more than a little and less than a lot of previous relationship experience.

ERIN ROGERS LEADS a workshop for people in southern California who feel that they are having trouble finding a healthy relationship. "What do you tell someone new you meet about your past?" Rogers asks the participants.

The answers range from lengthy and truthful disclosures to complete works of fiction to active omissions. "People feel like their relationship past is almost like a criminal record; if they reveal what's happened they will be less trusted and have trouble starting a new relationship.

"What I tell them, though, is they have to get past this used car mentality. You are not trying to hide the miles and roll back the odometer. Everybody has a past. Neither you nor anyone you meet is a brand-new person with no experiences."

Rogers asks her workshop participants to write their relationship history down—but only for themselves. When they have a firm grasp of their own full story, she talks them through relating that story to a potential partner.

"Step one is to accept your past. You can never explain where you've been and expect someone to understand and support your story if you don't accept it yourself. Step two is to figure out how to relate your past in a way that is both truthful and nonthreatening. You do not want to lie because if the new relationship works out, you will only have to deal with those lies down the road. But you also do not want to portray yourself in such a way that there will be no chance for the new relationship to work out."

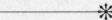

In studies asking people to rate their interest in dating another person, increasing that person's past number of sexual partners from zero up to four makes them sound more desirable. Each partner beyond five, however, makes the person sound less desirable. (Kenrick, Sundie, Nicastle, and Stone 2001)

98

It's for You—or It Isn't

We hear so many messages telling us what is expected and what is normal. Friends and family might mean well when they ask, "When are you going to get married?" or "When are you going to have children?" But their questions can come across as pressure to conform to some external standard. Your future, your goals, your relationships are not a means of answering critics. When and whether you do something are for you alone to decide. We cannot live our life seeking the acceptance of others because doing so will compromise our ability to gain acceptance from the most important source: ourselves.

"I'M OLD ENOUGH not to have to listen to anyone," says Roland, a retiree who tells people he's almost as old as the state of Arizona. "And it's a good thing, too. First they tell you what you have to do; then they tell you what you can't do."

Widowed ten years ago, Roland remembers being hurried along toward marriage when he was in his late twenties. And now his family wonders why he has a wedding date set for his marriage to Emma.

"I used to say I'm not getting married until I'm good and ready. And that's that. Now I say the same thing, except I am good and ready. I'm getting married because what I like about Emma can be summed up in two words: *practically everything*. I think she is a kind, understanding, loving person. She gives of herself for everyone, freely. She thinks of others. Very outgoing. She just loves people and to be around people."

Roland and Emma met at a Virginia senior recreation center. "We were sitting at the table in the cafeteria, and we just started talking," Roland says, laughing shyly. "And we became interested in each other." The moral of his story as Roland sees it: "When you find someone you think is swell, act. Until then, don't worry about it."

People who felt pressure from friends or family were 27 percent less likely to express satisfaction with their lack of a relationship if they were currently seeking one, and 12 percent less likely to express satisfaction with their relationship if they were currently seeing someone. (Barile 2001)

99

See the Horizon, Watch Your Step

R elationships are built on long-term values and short-term actions. You need to see the long-term goals and needs that your relationship will fulfill. This long-term perspective will give your relationship value to you in the moment, which is where you need to demonstrate, on a day-to-day, moment-to-moment basis, your dedication to a healthy relationship. As is the case with anything you really want in life, you need to see the long-term hope and the short-term need.

FAMED PHOTOGRAPHER Alfred Stieglitz was unhappy when his wife, painter Georgia O'Keeffe, kept talking about spending summers in the Southwest. He much preferred his family's retreat at Lake George in upstate New York. She did not. Finally, she decided to go on her own.

O'Keeffe told friends that her first summer in the Southwest was "bliss" and that she'd "never felt better in her life." But Stieglitz did not see it that way. He called it "maybe the most trying" experience of his life. He flooded her with letters. One day she received fifteen. But he kept busy and saw friends, and when she returned he told her about two new interests: flying a seaplane over the Hudson and playing classical music on his new Victrola. He never took her up on her offer to come join her in what she called "my faraway." But he did take a lot more photographs of her when she got back from that first trip. More than he had in years.

The notion of a marriage sabbatical—time away from one's partner to refresh oneself—has advocates among psychologists. "It's not for everyone," psychologist Penelope Sanders said. "If you don't have a burning desire to write or hike the Appalachian Trail or study in India, that's just fine. I'm not advocating that every married person take off. I'm just advocating that we broaden our ideas of what's possible in marriage.

"Whenever you do something alone and something hard, and you do it well, you can't help but feel really good about yourself and really good about life," Sanders said. "And those feelings spill over to your relationship."

It doesn't mean trouble in a marriage. Sanders thinks it means that a marriage is strong and encourages growth, individualism, renewal, the pursuit of dreams. "You're not leaving a marriage. What you're leaving is the day-to-day routine of married life.

"As long as we immerse ourselves in our families, we don't have to think about what we really want to do. We're always waiting. In many relationships people are there in the house, but the marriage is not alive in any way, shape, or form," Sanders said. "Physical closeness is not synonymous with emotional intimacy."

Sanders calls a marriage sabbatical "an amazing kind of long-term investment." It can strengthen a relationship, helping people feel closer to each other than ever before. Fulfilling this short-term need can improve the health of the relationship over the long term.

People in satisfying relationships were five times more likely to have a long-term perspective on their life, actively thinking about the long-term future instead of looking only at the short term. (Arriaga and Agnew 2001)

100

The Search for Perfection Is Endless

There is a difference between looking for something that is healthy and satisfying and looking for something that is perfect. The difference is that healthy and satisfying exist; perfect does not. Your relationship should contribute to your life and to the life of your partner. It should not be expected to provide you with someone who agrees with your every thought and preference or who can fill your every moment with joy. Seek fulfillment and you will find it; seek utopia and you will be looking forever.

"I DON'T THINK you'll ever really know a person unless you really have to share everything with them," said Christine, a computer programmer in Florida. She wondered what direction to take after moving in with her boyfriend. "I mean, on the one hand, it was like, 'Oh, my God, his feet smell!' and on the other hand, he seems to be a nice guy. But I didn't know if this was what I wanted forever."

They lived together for a year. They seemed to be happy. Then they happened to see the film *Indecent Proposal* on cable one night. After the movie, she asked him if he'd trade her in for a million dollars. He said not for one million, not for ten million.

"And I thought that was sweet. And I realized I just liked and loved him so much, I wanted to spend my life with him," she said. "I just knew he was the guy for me. Now, my parents thought I was too impulsive and that it wouldn't work out. But I didn't listen. I just followed my heart." They got married. They're still happy.

"Day to day, it's all about compromise," she said. "It's about giving in and saying you're sorry or dumb, as the case may be, and being sometimes brutally honest. Because love isn't about two puzzle pieces that fit together perfectly but about two people with similarities and differences and strengths and weaknesses."

People high in perfectionism, a hyperbelief in their own correctness and a desire to find a partner with similar traits, are 33 percent less likely to describe their relationship status as satisfying. (Flett, Hewitt, Shapiro, and Rayman 2002)

Sources

Acitelli, L., D. Kenny, and D. Weiner. 2001. "The Importance of Similarity and Understanding of Partners' Marital Ideals to Relationship Satisfaction." *Personal Relationships* 8:167–85.

Allen, S., and P. Webster. 2001. "When Wives Get Sick: Gender Role Attitude, Marital Happiness, and Husbands' Contribution to Household Labor." *Gender and Society* 15:898–916.

Alvaro, J. 2001. "An Interpersonal Forgiveness and Reconciliation Intervention: The Effect on Marital Intimacy." Ph.D. dissertation, New Orleans Baptist Theological Seminary.

Appleton, C., and E. Bohm. 2001. "Partners in Passage: The Experience of Marriage in Mid-Life." *Journal of Phenomenological Psychology* 32:41–70.

Arriaga, X., and C. Agnew. 2001. "Being Committed: Affective, Cognitive, and Conative Components of Relationship Commitment." *Personality and Social Psychology Bulletin* 27:1190–1203.

Arrindell, W., and F. Luteijn. 2000. "Similarity Between Intimate Partners for Personality Traits as Related to Individual Levels of Satisfaction with Life." *Personality and Individual Differences* 28:629–37.

Bachand, L., and S. Caron. 2001. "Ties That Bind: A Qualitative Study of Happy Long-Term Marriages." *Contemporary Family Therapy* 21:105–21.

Ball, L. 2000. "How Gender Differences Contribute to Divorce: A Retrospective Qualitative Study." Ph.D. dissertation, California School of Professional Psychology.

Barile, C. 2001. "The Never-Married, Caucasian, American Woman in Mid-Life as a Departure from the Stereotypes of the Old Maid Spinster." Ph.D. dissertation, Pacifica Graduate Institute.

Beach, S., D. Whitaker, D. Jones, and A. Tesser. 2001. "When Does Performance Feedback Prompt Complementarity in Romantic Relationships?" *Personal Relationships* 8:231–48.

Becker, P., and P. Moen. 1999. "Scaling Back: Dual-Earner Couples' Work-Family Strategies." *Journal of Marriage and the Family* 61:995–1007.

Berry, J., and E. Worthington. 2001. "Forgivingness, Relationship Quality, Stress While Imagining Relationship Events, and Physical and Mental Health." *Journal of Counseling Psychology* 48:447–55.

Blair, A. 2001. "Individuation, Love Styles, and Health-Related Quality of Life Among College Students." Ph.D. dissertation, University of Florida.

Bonds-Raacke, J., E. Bearden, N. Carriere, E. Anderson, and S. Nicks. 2001. "Engaging Distortions: Are We Idealizing Marriage?" *Journal of Psychology* 135:179–84.

Bosson, J., and W. Swann. 2001. "The Paradox of the Sincere Chameleon: Strategic Self-Verification in Close Relationships." In *Close Romantic Relationships: Maintenance and Enhancement,* edited by J. Harvey and A. Wenzel. Mahwah, NJ: Lawrence Erlbaum Associates.

Boyer-Pennington, M., J. Pennington, and C. Spink. 2001. "Students' Expectations and Optimism Toward Marriage as a Function of Parental Divorce." *Journal of Divorce and Remarriage* 34:71–87.

Broemer, P. 2001. "Ease of Recall Moderates the Impact of Relationship-Related Goals on Judgments of Interpersonal Closeness." *Journal of Experimental Social Psychology* 37:261–66.

Brown, S. 2000. "Union Transitions Among Cohabitors: The Significance of Relationship Assessments and Expectations." *Journal of Marriage and the Family* 62:833–46.

Bumpass, L., and J. Sweet. 2001. "Marriage, Divorce, and Intergenerational Relationships." In *The Well-Being of Children and Families,* edited by A. Thornton. Ann Arbor: University of Michigan Press.

Burland, A. 2001. "Attachment and Emotion Regulation in Dating Relationships: Exposure and Reactivity to Daily Appraisals of Partner Behavior." Ph.D. dissertation, University of Delaware.

Bush, H., R. Williams, M. Lean, and A. Anderson. 2001. "Body Image and Weight Consciousness Among South Asian, Italian, and General Population Women in Britain." *Appetite* 37:207–15.

Buss, D., T. Shackelford, L. Kirkpatrick, and R. Larsen. 2001. "A Half Century of Mate Preferences: The Cultural Evolution of Values." *Journal of Marriage and the Family* 63:491–503.

Buunk, B., and W. Mutsaers. 1999. "The Nature of the Relationship Between Remarried Individuals and Former Spouses and Its Impact on Marital Satisfaction." *Journal of Family Psychology* 13:165–74.

Campbell, L., J. Simpson, D. Kashy, and W. Rholes. 2001. "Attachment Orientations, Dependence, and Behavior in a Stressful Situation: An Application of the Actor-Partner Interdependence Model." *Journal of Social and Personal Relationships* 18:821–43.

Carrere, S., K. Buehlman, J. Gottman, J. Coan, and L. Ruckstuhl. 2000. "Predicting Marital Stability and Divorce in Newlywed Couples." *Journal of Family Psychology* 14:42–58.

Carsten, K. 2001. "Enhancing Satisfaction Through Downward Comparison: The Role of Relational Discontent and Individual Differences in Social Comparison Orientation." *Journal of Experimental Social Psychology* 37:452–67.

Cauffield, C., J. Moye, and L. Travis. 1999. "Long-Term Marital Conflict: Antecedents to and Consequences for Discharge Planning." *Clinical Gerontologist* 20:82–86.

Caughlin, J., and T. Huston. 2002. "A Contextual Analysis of the Association Between Demand/Withdraw and Marital Satisfaction." *Personal Relationships* 9:95–119.

Chou, K., and I. Chi. 2001. "Stressful Life Events and Depressive Symptoms: Social Support and Sense of Control as Mediators or Moderators?" *International Journal of Aging and Human Development* 52:155–71.

Clements, R., and C. Swensen. 2000. "Commitment to One's Spouse as a Predictor of Marital Quality Among Older Couples." *Current Psychology* 19:110–19.

Cohan, C., and S. Cole. 2002. "Life Course Transitions and Natural Disaster: Marriage, Birth, and Divorce Following Hurricane Hugo." *Journal of Family Psychology* 16:14–25.

Cole, M. 2000. "The Experience of Never-Married Women in Their Thirties Who Desire Marriage and Children." Ph.D. dissertation, Institute for Clinical Social Work.

Collins, N., and B. Feeney. 2000. "A Safe Haven: An Attachment Theory Perspective on Support Seeking and Caregiving in Intimate Relationships." *Journal of Personality and Social Psychology* 78:1053–73.

Conway, C. 2000. "Using the Crucial Cs to Explore Gender Roles with Couples." *Journal of Individual Psychology* 56:495–501.

Cox, D. 2001. "'Smile, Honey, Our Church Is Watching': Identity and Role Conflict in the Pastoral Marriage." Ph.D. dissertation, University of South Florida.

Davis, J., and C. Rusbult. 2001. "Attitude Alignment in Close Relationships." *Journal of Personality and Social Psychology* 81:65–84.

De Koning, E., and R. Weiss. 2002. "The Relational Humor Inventory: Functions of Humor in Close Relationships." *American Journal of Family Therapy* 30:1–18.

Diener, E., C. Gohn, E. Eunkook, and S. Oishi. 2000. "Similarity of the Relations Between Marital Status and Subjective Well-Being Across Cultures." *Journal of Cross-Cultural Psychology* 31:419–36.

Drigotas, S., C. Rusbult, and J. Verette. 1999. "Level of Commitment, Mutuality of Commitment, and Couple Well-Being." *Personal Relationships* 6:389–409.

Dufore, S. 2000. "Marital Similarity, Marital Interaction, and Couples' Shared View of Their Marriage." Ph.D. dissertation, Syracuse University.

Dugosh, J. 2001. "Effects of Relationship Threat and Ambiguity on Empathic Accuracy in Dating Couples." Ph.D. dissertation, University of Texas at Arlington.

Ebesu Hubbard, A. 2001. "Conflict Between Relationally Uncertain Romantic Partners: The Influence of Relational Responsiveness and Empathy." *Communication Monographs* 68:400–414.

Eldridge, K. 2001. "Demand-Withdraw Communication During Marital Conflict: Relationship Satisfaction and Gender Role Considerations." Ph.D. dissertation, University of California, Los Angeles.

Elizabeth, V. 2000. "Cohabitation, Marriage, and the Unruly Consequences of Difference." *Gender and Society* 14:87–110.

Erera, P., and K. Fredriksen. 1999. "Lesbian Stepfamilies: A Unique Family Structure." *Families in Society* 80:263–70.

Fahrenkamp, E. 2001. "Age, Gender, and Perceived Social Support of Married and Never-Married Persons as Predictors of Self-Esteem." Ph.D. dissertation, Texas A&M University.

Felmlee, D. 2001. "From Appealing to Appalling: Disenchantment with a Romantic Partner." *Sociological Perspectives* 44:263–80.

Fisher, H. 2000. "Lust, Attraction, Attachment: Biology and Evolution of the Three Primary Emotion Systems for Mating, Reproduction, and Parenting." *Journal of Sex Education and Therapy* 25:96–104.

Fitness, J. 2001. "Emotional Intelligence and Intimate Relationships." In *Emotional Intelligence in Everyday Life: A Scientific Inquiry*, edited by J. Ciarrochi and J. Forgas. New York: Psychology Press.

Fitzgerald, T. 1999. "Who Marries Whom? Attitudes and Behavior in Marital Partner Selection." Ph.D. dissertation, University of Colorado.

Flett, G., P. Hewitt, B. Shapiro, and J. Rayman. 2002. "Perfectionism, Beliefs, and Adjustment in Dating Relationships." *Current Psychology* 20:289–311.

Flora, J., and C. Segrin. 1999. "Social Skills Are Associated with Satisfaction in Close Relationships." *Psychological Reports* 84:803–4.

———. 2001. "The Association Between Accounts of Relationship Development Events and Relational and Personal Well-Being." In *Attribution, Communication Behavior, and Close Relationships*, edited by V. Manusov and J. Harvey. New York: Cambridge University Press.

Fowers, B. 2001. "The Limits of Technical Concept of a Good Marriage: Exploring the Role of Virtue in Communication Skills." *Journal of Marital and Family Therapy* 27:327–40.

Fowers, B., E. Lyons, K. Montel, and N. Shaked. 2001. "Positive Illusions About Marriage Among Married and Single Individuals." *Journal of Family Psychology* 15:95–109.

Freeman, L., D. Templer, and C. Hill. 1999. "The Relationship Between Adult Happiness and Self-Appraised Childhood Happiness and Events." *Journal of Genetic Psychology* 160:46–54.

Gagne, F., and J. Lydon. 2001. "Mind-Set and Relationship Illusions: The Moderating Effects of Domain Specificity and Relationship Commitment." *Personality and Social Psychology Bulletin* 27:1144–55.

Gilbert, L., and S. Walker. 2001. "Contemporary Marriage." In *The New Handbook of Psychotherapy and Counseling with Men,* edited by G. Brooks and G. Glenn. San Francisco: Jossey-Bass.

Goldscheider, F. 1999. "Men's Changing Family Relationships." In *Couples in Conflict,* edited by A. Booth and A. Crouter. State College: Pennsylvania State University.

Goodman, C. 1999. "Reciprocity of Social Support in Long-Term Marriage." *Journal of Mental Health and Aging* 5:341–57.

Gottman, J., and R. Levenson. 2000. "The Timing of Divorce: Predicting When a Couple Will Divorce over a Fourteen-Year Period." *Journal of Marriage and the Family* 62:737–45.

Greeff, A. 2000. "Characteristics of Families That Function Well." *Journal of Family Issues* 21:948–62.

Greeff, A., and T. De Bruyne. 2000. "Conflict Management Style and Marital Satisfaction." *Journal of Sex and Marital Therapy* 26:321–34.

Hairston, R. 2001. "Predicting Marital Satisfaction Among African American Couples." Ph.D. dissertation, Seattle Pacific University.

Hannon, M. 2001. "Perpetrator Behavior and Forgiveness in Close Relationships." Ph.D. dissertation, University of North Carolina.

Harris, K. 2001. "The Psychophysiology of Marital Interaction: Differential Effects of Support and Conflict." Ph.D. dissertation, University of Oregon.

Herold, E., and R. Milhausen. 1999. "Dating Preferences of University Women: An Analysis of the Nice Guy Stereotype." *Journal of Sex and Marital Therapy* 25:333–43.

Hetsroni, A. 2000. "Choosing a Mate in Television Dating Games: The Influence of Setting, Culture, and Gender." *Sex Roles* 42:83–106.

Hilfer, M. 1999. "Examination of Altruistic Behavior as a Means of Attenuating Marital Blame." Ph.D. dissertation, Ohio State University.

Honeycutt, J. 1999. "Typological Differences in Predicting Marital Happiness from Oral History Behaviors and Imagined Interactions." *Communication Monographs* 66:276–91.

Housker, J. 2001. "Houston's Model of Guided Imagery Combined with Music: Strengthening Couples' Relationships." Ph.D. dissertation, University of South Dakota.

Huston, T. 2000. "The Social Ecology of Marriage and Other Intimate Unions." *Journal of Marriage and the Family* 62:298–319.

Huston, T., J. Caughlin, R. Houts, S. Smith, and L. George. 2001. "The Connubial Crucible: Newlywed Years as Predictors of Marital Delight, Distress, and Divorce." *Journal of Personality and Social Psychology* 80:237–52.

Jabs, C. 2000. "Depression and Marital Interaction: An Analysis of Systemic Patterns of Marital Communication." Ph.D. dissertation, University of Chicago.

Jackman Cram, S. 2000. "Depression in Marriage: An Investigation of Problem-Solving Behavior and Marital Cognition." Ph.D. dissertation, University of Calgary.

Jagger, E. 2001. "Marketing Molly and Melville: Dating in a Postmodern, Consumer Society." *Sociology* 35:39–57.

Jansezian, K. 2001. "Gender Differences in Perceived Love, Empathy, Relationship Satisfaction, Family Influence, and Importance of Money and Material Things Among Individuals in Current Dating or Marital Interracial or Intraracial Relationships." Ph.D. dissertation, California School of Professional Psychology.

Ji, J. 2001. "Linkages Between Maternal Influence and Adult Children's Marital Quality." Ph.D. dissertation, Mississippi State University.

Johnson, K. 1999. "Love at the Launching Stage: Predicting Expectations of Marital Endurance." Ph.D. dissertation, Barry University.

Johnson, M., B. Karney, R. Rogge, and T. Bradbury. 2001. "The Role of Marital Behavior in the Longitudinal Association Between Attributions and Marital

Quality." In *Attribution, Communication Behavior, and Close Relationships,* edited by V. Manusov and J. Harvey. New York: Cambridge University Press.

Juang, L., and R. Silbereisen. 2001. "Family Transitions for Young Adult Women." *American Behavioral Scientist* 44:1899–1917.

Julien, D., N. Tremblay, I. Belanger, M. Dube, J. Begin, and D. Bouthillier. 2000. "Interaction Structure of Husbands' and Wives' Disclosure of Marital Conflict to Their Respective Best Friend." *Journal of Family Psychology* 14:286–303.

Kalmijn, M., and H. Flap. 2001. "Assortative Meeting and Mating: Unintended Consequences of Organized Settings for Partner Choices." *Social Forces* 79:1289–1312.

Karney, B., and T. Bradbury. 2000. "Attributions in Marriage: State or Trait? A Growth Curve Analysis." *Journal of Personality and Social Psychology* 78:295–309.

Karney, B., and N. Frye. 2002. " 'But We've Been Getting Better Lately': Comparing Prospective and Retrospective Views of Relationship Development." *Journal of Personality and Social Psychology* 82:222–38.

Kelly, A., and J. Carter. 2001. "Dealing with Secrets." In *Coping with Stress: Effective People and Processes,* edited by C. Snyder. New York: Oxford University Press.

Kenrick, D., J. Sundie, L. Nicastle, and G. Stone. 2001. "Can One Ever Be Too Wealthy or Too Chaste? Searching for Non-linearities in Mate Judgment." *Journal of Personality and Social Psychology* 80:462–71.

Klute, M., A. Crouter, A. Sayer, and S. McHale. 2002. "Occupational Self-Direction, Values, and Egalitarian Relationships: A Study of Dual-Earner Couples." *Journal of Marriage and Family* 64:139–51.

Knobloch, L., D. Solomon, and M. Cruz. 2001. "The Role of Relationship Development and Attachment in the Experience of Romantic Jealousy." *Personal Relationships* 8:205–24.

Knox, D., and M. Zusman. 2001. "Marrying a Man with 'Baggage': Implications for Second Wives." *Journal of Divorce and Remarriage* 35:67–79.

Koehne, K. 2000. "The Relationship Between Relational Commitment, Spousal Intimacy, and Religiosity and Marital Satisfaction." Ph.D. dissertation, University of Tennessee.

Kulik, L. 2001. "The Impact of Men's and Women's Retirement on Marital Relations: A Comparative Analysis." *Journal of Women and Aging* 13:21–37.

Kurdek, L. 1999. "The Nature and Predictors of the Trajectory of Change in Marital Quality for Husbands and Wives over the First Ten Years of Marriage." *Developmental Psychology* 35:1283–96.

Lawrence, T. 2001. "Secure Base Behaviors and Mental Representations of Attachment in Early Marriage." Ph.D. dissertation, State University of New York at Stony Brook.

Lester, D. 1999. "Social Correlates of Divorce Rates." *Perceptual and Motor Skills* 88:1330.

LeSure-Lester, G. 2001. "Dating Competence, Social Assertion, and Social Anxiety Among College Students." *College Student Journal* 35:317–20.

Levine, S. 2000. "Gender Differences in Loneliness and Marital Quality in Young Married Couples." Ph.D. dissertation, California School of Professional Psychology.

Lockhart, A. 2000. "Perceived Influence of a Disney Fairy Tale on Beliefs About Romantic Love and Marriage." Ph.D. dissertation, California School of Professional Psychology.

Lord, C. 2000. "Stability and Change on Interactional Behavior in Early Marriage." Ph.D. dissertation, State University of New York at Stony Brook.

Loveless, A. 2000. "Paired Conceptions of Morality and Happiness as Factors in Marital Happiness." Ph.D. dissertation, Brigham Young University.

Ludlow, L., and R. Alvarez-Salvat. 2001. "Spillover in the Academy: Marriage Stability and Faculty Evaluations." *Journal of Personal Evaluation in Education* 15:111–19.

Ludwig, K. 2000. "Responses to Dissatisfaction: An Integrative Analysis of Change Attempts and Relationship Quality." Ph.D. dissertation, Auburn University.

MacDonald, T., and M. Ross. 1999. "Assessing the Accuracy of Predictions About Dating Relationships: How and Why Do Lovers' Predictions Differ from Those Made by Observers?" *Personality and Social Psychology Bulletin* 25:1417–29.

Maguire, M. 1999. "Occupational Self-Direction, Values, and Egalitarian Relationships in Dual-Earner Couples." Ph.D. dissertation, Pennsylvania State University.

Marks, S., T. Huston, E. Johnson, and S. MacDermid. 2001. "Role Balance Among White Married Couples." *Journal of Marriage and the Family* 63:1083–98.

McFadden, J. 2001. "Intercultural Marriage and Family: Beyond the Racial Divide." *Family Journal* 9:39–42.

Medora, N., J. Larson, N. Hortacsu, and D. Parul. 2002. "Perceived Attitudes Toward Romanticism." *Journal of Comparative Family Studies* 33:155–78.

Murray, S., and J. Holmes. 1999. "The Mental Ties That Bind: Cognitive Structures That Predict Relationship Resilience." *Journal of Personality and Social Psychology* 77:1228–44.

Murray, S., J. Holmes, D. Dolderman, and D. Griffin. 2000. "What the Motivated Mind Sees: Comparing Friends' Perspectives to Married Partners' Views of Each Other." *Journal of Experimental Social Psychology* 36:600–620.

Murray, S., J. Holmes, and D. Griffin. 2000. "Self-Esteem and the Quest for Felt Security: How Perceived Regard Regulates Attachment Processes." *Journal of Personality and Social Psychology* 78:478–98.

Murray, S., J. Holmes, D. Griffin, G. Bellavia, and P. Rose. 2001. "The Mismeasure of Love: How Self-Doubt Contaminates Relationship Beliefs." *Personality and Social Psychology Bulletin* 27:423–36.

Nardi, R. 2000. "Commitment to Emotional Relationships Between Men and Women: The Differences and Implications of Modern Marriage." Ph.D. dissertation, The Union Institute.

Nock, S. 2001. "The Marriages of Equally Dependent Spouses." *Journal of Family Issues* 22:755–75.

O'Leary, J. 2000. "College Students' Role Expectations in Marriage." Ph.D. dissertation, Indiana University of Pennsylvania.

Oner, B. 2001. "Factors Predicting Future Time Orientation for Romantic Relationships with the Opposite Sex." *Journal of Psychology* 135:430–38.

Orrego, V. 2000. "Values and Attitudes Toward Interracial Marriage: An Examination of the Value Expressive Function." Ph.D. dissertation, Michigan State University.

Pallen, R. 2001. "Intimacy, Need Fulfillment, and Violence in Marital Relationships." Ph.D. dissertation, University of Arkansas.

Palmer-Daley, J. 2001. "Imagination: The Stuff That Love Is Made Of." Ph.D. dissertation, Pacifica Graduate Institute.

Pals, J. 1999. "Identity Consolidation in Early Adulthood: Relations with Ego-Resiliency, the Context of Marriage, and Personality Changes." *Journal of Personality* 67:295–329.

Pape, A. 2001. "Conflict Resolution Satisfaction: A Study of Satisfied Marriages Across Sixteen Domains of Marital Conflict." Ph.D. dissertation, Texas Women's University.

Philpot, C. 2001. "Someday My Prince Will Come." In *Casebook for Integrating Family Therapy,* edited by S. McDaniel and D. Lusterman. Washington, DC: American Psychological Association.

Porter, G. 2001. "Workaholics as High-Performance Employees: The Intersection of Workplace and Family Relationship Problems." In *High-Performing Families: Causes, Consequences, and Clinical Solutions,* edited by B. Robinson and N. Chase. Washington, DC: American Counseling Association.

Prescott, C., and K. Kendler. 2001. "Associations Between Marital Status and Alcohol Consumption in a Longitudinal Study of Female Twins." *Journal of Studies on Alcohol* 62:589–604.

Presser, H. 2000. "Nonstandard Work Schedules and Marital Instability." *Journal of Marriage and the Family* 62:93–110.

Price, D. 2002. *Finding a Lover for Life: A Gay Man's Guide to Finding a Lasting Relationship.* New York: Haworth Press.

Protinsky, H., and L. Coward. 2001. "Developmental Lessons of Seasoned Marital and Family Therapists: A Qualitative Investigation." *Journal of Marital and Family Therapy* 27:375–84.

Roberts, N., and R. Levenson. 2001. "The Remains of the Workday: Impact of Job Stress and Exhaustion on Marital Interaction in Police Couples." *Journal of Marriage and the Family* 63:1052–67.

Rogers, S., and P. Amato. 2000. "Have Changes in Gender Relations Affected Marital Quality?" *Social Forces* 79:731–53.

Roloff, M., K. Soule, and C. Carey. 2001. "Reasons for Remaining in a Relationship and Responses to Relational Transgressions." *Journal of Social and Personal Relationships* 18:362–85.

Romero-Medina, A. 2001. "Sex-Equal Stable Marriages." *Theory and Decision* 50:197–212.

Ruef, A. 2001. "Empathy in Long-Term Marriage: Behavioral and Physiological Correlates." Ph.D. dissertation, University of California, Berkeley.

Saiz, C. 2001. "Teaching Couples Communication and Problem-Solving Skills." Ph.D. dissertation, University of Denver.

Sanchez, L., and C. Cager. 2000. "Hard Living, Perceived Entitlement to a Great Marriage, and Marital Dissolution." *Journal of Marriage and the Family* 62:708–22.

Savin-Williams, R., and K. Esterberg. 2000. "Lesbian, Gay, and Bisexual Families." In *Handbook of Family Diversity,* edited by D. Demo and K. Allen. New York: Oxford University Press.

Schneewind, K., and A. Gerhard. 2002. "Relationship Personality, Conflict Resolution, and Marital Satisfaction in the First Five Years of Marriage." *Family Relations* 51:63–71.

Schneider, J. 2000. "A Qualitative Study of Cybersex Participants: Gender Differences, Recovery Issues, and Implications for Therapists." *Sexual Addiction and Compulsivity* 7:249–78.

Schwartz, R. 2000. *Marriage in Motion: The Natural Ebb and Flow of Lasting Relationships.* Cambridge, MA: Perseus Publishing.

Shebilske, L. 2000. "Affective Quality, Leisure Time, and Marital Satisfaction: A Thirteen-Year Longitudinal Study." Ph.D. dissertation, University of Texas.

Skaldeman, P., and H. Montgomery. 1999. "Interpretational Incongruence of Value-Profiles: Perception of Own and Partner's Values in Married and Divorced Couples." *Journal of Social Behavior and Personality* 14:345–65.

Smith, H. 2000. "Marital Satisfaction and Locus of Control in Dual-Earner Couples: An Analysis of Current Trends." Ph.D. dissertation, University of Connecticut.

Solomon, D., and L. Knobloch. 2001. "Relationship Uncertainty, Partner Interference, and Intimacy Within Dating Relationships." *Journal of Social and Personal Relationships* 18:804–20.

South, S., and K. Crowder. 2000. "The Declining Significance of Neighborhoods? Marital Transitions in Community Context." *Social Forces* 78:1067–99.

Sprecher, S., and D. Felmlee. 2000. "Romantic Partners' Perceptions of Social Network Attributes with the Passage of Time and Relationship Transitions." *Personal Relationships* 7:325–40.

Stewart, S., H. Stinnett, and L. Rosenfeld. 2000. "Sex Differences in Desired Characteristics of Short-Term and Long-Term Relationship Partners." *Journal of Social and Personal Relationships* 17:843–53.

Sullivan, K. 2001. "Understanding the Relationship Between Religiosity and Marriage: An Investigation of the Immediate and Longitudinal Effects of Religiosity on Newlywed Couples." *Journal of Family Psychology* 15:610–26.

Sweeney, M. 2002. "Remarriage and the Nature of Divorce: Does It Matter Which Spouse Chose to Leave?" *Journal of Family Issues* 23:410–40.

Symmonds-Mueth, J. 2000. "Adult Males: Marital Satisfaction and General Life Contentment Across the Life Cycle." Ph.D. dissertation, University of Missouri, St. Louis.

Szinovacz, M., and A. Schaffer. 2000. "Effects of Retirement on Marital Conflict Tactics." *Journal of Family Issues* 21:367–89.

Takeuchi, S. 2000. "If I Don't Look Good, You Don't Look Good? Toward a New Matching Theory of Interpersonal Attraction Based on the Behavioral and the Social Exchange Principles." Ph.D. dissertation, Washington State University.

Taylor, D. 2001. "Weaving Modern-Day Wives' Tales: Women Redefining Wifehood." Ph.D. dissertation, Texas Tech University.

Thomas, J. 1999. "Relationship Efficacy: The Prediction of Goal Attainment by Dating Couples." Ph.D. dissertation, University of Maryland.

Thornton, A., and L. Young-DeMarco. 2001. "Four Decades of Trends in Attitudes Toward Family Issues in the United States." *Journal of Marriage and the Family* 63:1009–37.

Timmer, S., and J. Veroff. 2000. "Family Ties and the Discontinuity of Divorce in Black and White Newlywed Couples." *Journal of Marriage and the Family* 62:349–61.

Turner, H., and R. Turner. 1999. "Gender, Social Status, and Emotional Reliance." *Journal of Health and Social Behavior* 40:360–73.

Vaughn, L. 2001. "The Relationship Between Marital Satisfaction Levels Associated with Participation in the Free and Hope-Focused Marital Enrichment Program." Ph.D. dissertation, Regent University.

Vaughn, M. 2000. "Creating 'Maneuvering Room': A Grounded Theory of Language and Therapist Influence in Marriage and Family Therapy." Ph.D. dissertation, Texas Tech University.

Vinograde, D. 2001. "Black and White Heterosexual Women's Marital and Same-Sex Best Friend Relationships, and the Contributions of Entitlement, Relationship Equality, and Relationship Intimacy to Well-Being." Ph.D. dissertation, Adelphi University.

Voss, K., D. Markiewicz, and A. Doyle. 1999. "Friendship, Marriage, and Self-Esteem." *Journal of Social and Personal Relationships* 16:103–22.

Wall, B. 2000. "What Keeps Unhappy Couples Together? A Qualitative and Theoretical Exploration." Ph.D. dissertation, Iowa State University.

Ward, M. 2002. "Does Television Exposure Affect Emerging Adults' Attitudes and Assumptions About Sexual Relationships?" *Journal of Youth and Adolescence* 31:1–15.

Watson, D., B. Hubbard, and D. Wiese. 2000. "General Traits of Personality and Affectivity as Predictors of Satisfaction in Intimate Relationships: Evidence from Self and Partner Ratings." *Journal of Personality* 68:413–49.

———. 2000. "Self-Other Agreement in Personality and Affectivity: The Role of Acquaintanceship, Trait Visibility, and Assumed Similarity." *Journal of Personality and Social Psychology* 78:465–558.

Weigel, D., and D. Ballard-Reisch. 1999. "The Influence of Marital Duration and the Use of Relationship Maintenance Behaviors." *Communication Reports* 12:59–70.

Werner, E., and R. Smith. 2001. *Journeys from Childhood to Midlife: Risk, Resilience, and Recovery.* Ithaca, NY: Cornell University Press.

Wiener, C. 1999. "Patterns of Friendship and Interpersonal Process in Marriage." Ph.D. dissertation, Adelphi University.

Witcher, B. 2000. "The Effect of Power on Relationships and on Individuals." Ph.D. dissertation, University of North Carolina.

Wu, P. 2001. "Analysis of the Effects of Marriage Encounter as a Form of Family Life Education." Ph.D. dissertation, Claremont Graduate University.

Yogev, S. 2002. *For Better or for Worse . . . But Not for Lunch: Making Marriage Work in Retirement.* New York: McGraw-Hill.

Zink, D. 2000. "The Enduring Marriages of Adult Children of Divorce." Ph.D. dissertation, St. Louis University.

Acknowledgments

It has been a pleasure to work with Gideon Weil and the staff of Harper San Francisco and Sandy Choron, my agent. I thank them for their efforts and their enthusiasm and for helping me to make this book a more useful tool for readers.

THE
SIMPLE SCIENCE OF A GREAT LIFE

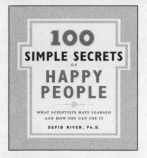

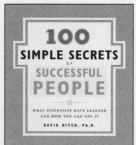

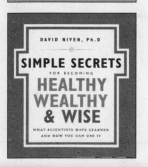

This bestselling series of scientifically based advice offers practical guidance on the most important aspects of our lives—happiness, success, relationships, and health. With close to a million copies sold, the Simple Secrets series takes the most valuable scientific research and delivers it in fun, easily digestible findings complete with real-world examples that people can use in their daily lives.

**100 SIMPLE SECRETS
OF HAPPY PEOPLE**
ISBN 0-06-115791-0

**100 SIMPLE SECRETS
OF SUCCESSFUL PEOPLE**
ISBN 0-06-115793-7

**365 SIMPLE SECRETS FOR BECOMING
HEALTHY, WEALTHY, AND WISE**
ISBN 0-06-085881-8

Now available in your bookstore.